Beat Fear:

The Science of Overcoming, Managing, and Using Fear to Live on Your Own Terms and Break Free of your Mental Prison

By Patrick King
Social Interaction Specialist and
Conversation Coach
www.PatrickKingConsulting.com

Table of Contents

Introduction

One of the funniest moments of my life was when my brother fell into the deep end of the local swimming pool. Of course, I was a young boy, and I thought it was hilarious to watch him scream and flail like one of those inflatable tube men you might see in front of a car dealership.

My parents didn't think it was so funny, and luckily they were on hand and jumped in to drag my brother to safety before any harm was done. I was too young to understand that neither my brother nor I could swim and that I would have fared even worse than him had I been the one to fall.

Even though my brother was fished out of the water before his head was even completely wet, he ended up carrying a subconscious fear with him for years afterward. On trips to the beach, he would stay with the towels and chairs while everyone else splashed each other with the salty ocean water, insisting that he wanted to safeguard our belongings. It wasn't until the senior year of high school that he had to come face to face with his fear, because the high school we attended had a swimming requirement. If you couldn't swim 100 meters and tread water for 60 seconds, you couldn't graduate.

Of course, for my brother, the first obstacle to overcome was to get in the water in the first place! Informed by the principal that there were absolutely no exceptions to be made, my parents grappled with how to approach this seemingly irrational fear—though actually quite rational if you consider his experiences.

My father, ever the tinkerer, read up on something he called *exposure therapy*. The rest of us had no idea what he was talking about, but we weren't in a situation to say otherwise, so we just followed his lead.

It turns out, the ways my brother perceived water went far deeper than avoiding pools, the ocean, or getting on boats. In fact, he felt an immense amount of psychological stress and anxiety whenever he was near a body of water that he didn't feel 100% safe near. Phrased another way, he felt discomfort whenever he was near water that had the possibility of killing him, like when it could cover his face and he was powerless to do anything about it.

Of course, in literal terms, he should be terrified by bowls of soup and shallow puddles after rainfall—but how was he going to use exposure therapy to deal with learning to swim?

They started slowly as I watched from the side. That first night, my father filled the bathtub up to the top and had my brother submerge himself to his waist. That was good for day one. The next day, he submerged himself up to his neck for about two seconds. The third day, he made it up to seven seconds.

That weekend we had another beach trip, but the purpose was far different than ever before. It was the same type of process, and each hour, my brother ventured another few inches into the water. At the end of the day, he could stand to be in chest-deep water—if my father was in striking distance. A couple of weeks later, he was floating in the ocean with his toes not being able to touch the ground. You might be able to see where this is going.

He ended up passing his swimming requirement and graduating high school, and I got a front row seat to one of the premiere ways to influence someone's behavior and make a lasting change despite the crushing specter of simple fear.

What is the role of fear in our lives?

It certainly doesn't seem to do us any favors, and often it seems like we would be better off if our fear receptors were simply severed. The truth is, much of what keeps us back in life isn't because of our ability or our talent—it's our perception of our ability, which is inexorably tied to fear. The fears of failure, fear itself, rejection, and judgment are things very few of us can escape.

So what do we make of fear? It's not a matter of making it vanish—it's a matter of *managing and understanding* it. Fear will always have a strong purpose in our lives, and when you can listen to it yet not allow it to dictate your decisions, that's how you **beat fear**.

Chapter 1. "Formidoectomy"

It's common practice for people to have various surgical procedures to improve health and quality of life. Many people opt for elective surgeries to assist with weight loss, sagging body parts, and poor eyesight. Gastric sleeve, plastic surgery, facelifts, tummy tucks, and liposuction are all ways people try to improve physical appearance.

What about mental constitution?

Today I want to introduce you to a new procedure: the *formidoectomy*. This new term is based on the Latin word *formido*, which means fear, fearfulness, dread, and panic, and the Greek suffix *ectomy*, which means the act of cutting out. The meaning is simply cutting out fear, but the procedure is time-consuming, scary in itself, and you aren't able to simply sew yourself back up immediately.

Unlike a surgical procedure, the formidoectomy does not include a hospital stay or follow-up medications. It involves developing a new mindset, adjusting self-talk, identifying fears, and taking daily steps to make the real and lasting changes you want to see. It is about learning to live fearlessly, even when that feels terrifying.

The purpose of this book is to help you through *your* formidoectomy. There's no magic pill and no surgical operation, but if you believe fear is holding you back, then this is just the procedure you need.

What Is Fear?

As a child, fear seems like an easy foe to conquer. Afraid of the dark? Overcome fear with a nightlight.

Afraid of deep water? Floaties and two weeks of swimming lessons later, and what was once feared is suddenly loved.

Monsters in the closet? A quick spritz of "Monster B Gone" before bed does the trick (and smells a lot like honeysuckle or lilac).

What *is* fear? True fear is more complex and difficult to overcome. A child who is raised in an abusive home does not escape night terrors by saying a brief prayer to a resin guardian angel above his bed. The spouse of a terminally ill patient does not just pull on the boot straps and feel brave. Fear is a natural part of life, but when fear becomes the controlling factor in life, that is when it needs to be eliminated. That is when it is time for the formidoectomy.

Fear is what keeps us from doing what we want. It is the obstacle in front of our goals, and it is the little voice inside our heads telling us every bad thing that can happen, no matter the probability. It can be paralyzing. Facing mortgages, insurance bills, college tuition costs, and car payments after the loss of a job can put people in a position of not having any idea where to turn or what to do first. It can be terrifying to imagine the worst-case scenario when a loved one receives a serious medical diagnosis.

Fear seizes control of our minds because it is predicated on the avoidance of pain and, to a lesser degree, the pursuit of pleasure. In fact, in a recent study, Todd Kashdan discovered that people are willing to pay more money to avoid fear than to experience happiness. To be happy, people are willing to pay $79.06, while to avoid fear, people are willing to up the price to $83.27.

As a species, we instinctively seek pleasure and avoid pain. Unfortunately, we can't just pay a price and be rid of our fears like magic. As you read this book, consider the question, "Am I willing to pay the cost to cut fear out of my life?" The costs, sweat, and tears might be substantial, but are they comparable to what your fears are causing you to miss?

Fear is often not about the actual pain or consequences themselves; it's everything that leads up to it, including the anticipation and uncertainty. A shot never hurts quite as much as we expect it to, but the fear of the shot can send even the strongest people to their knees. It is the fear we despise, because we do not control it or its consequences.

Likewise, our fears are often far more frightening than reality could ever be. Humans may be the only creatures with the ability to conjure up the worst-case scenario in even the most benign situations. A father is ready to arm the troops when his daughter is 20 minutes past curfew only to receive a text saying the movie ran late and she is on the way home. A coworker convinces herself the slight crack in her voice when she met the client immediately sent the deal to another agency. Fearing the worst will come true is the human curse, yet so often those fears are unfounded.

What is fear? Fear is often not a reflection of reality, and yet we take it far more seriously than near certainties.

Have you ever driven on an icy road and suddenly realized your tires are skidding? Even if it is just for a brief moment, that loss-of-control feeling is unmistakable: heart races, breath stops, palms become drenched.

One of the worst aspects of fear is it brings a feeling of being out of control. People don't imagine only one worst-case scenario—their imaginations do their best to one-up the previous scenario with horror and terror. While it is sometimes possible to recognize the worst-case scenario will not become reality, there are plenty of *less than the worst but still terrible* options upon which to dwell. It's hard to feel like you have any semblance of control when you are potentially staring at your life crumbling before your eyes. We lose any semblance of logic and rational thinking.

Health-care scares are notorious for making people feel out of control. Finding a lump during a monthly self-exam can ignite an imagination tailspin. Even with a quick call to the doctor, there is a period of time that feels as if no one is really in control. There is no plan of action, no expert opinion, no options to compare. Until there is at the very least an appointment, a scan, or a consultation, the problem feels like a semi-truck without a driver on a dark, curvy road.

For many of us, it is the unknown consequences that create the fear: the diagnosis could be fatal; the recovery could be painful; the insurance payments might not cover the treatments; the technology may not be set up correctly; the plan may be too aggressive (or too conservative); the client might be offended by the graphics.

The constant rumination of that which is beyond control increases the level of stress. The higher that stress level reaches, the more difficult it is to think straight and to develop rational plans. It is normal and fine to fear the cancer; it is not mentally or physically healthy, though, to worry over every little detail to the point you cannot make good decisions.

What is fear? It has the destructive power to hijack your brain for its nefarious purposes and won't let go until far too late.

The Many Faces of Fear

As stated earlier, feeling afraid during a major crisis is natural; however, ignoring the day-to-day chronic variety of free-floating anxiety is no healthier than ignoring those heavy, life-altering difficult issues.

Constant worry about the future makes it impossible to enjoy the present. Anxiety robs people of the joy life experiences can bring. Insecurity eliminates the desire and courage to step out, take risks, and try new things. For many, it is the small everyday fears that eat away at our physical and emotional health rather than the monumental traumas. It is like a hazy cloud that starts accumulating around you—you don't notice its presence until it is already considerable in size.

It is important to gain control in a crisis situation like a health scare, a terrorist attack, a near-fatal accident, or a job loss. It is easy to forget that other, less dramatic fears can take their toll on emotional health as well. No one would judge parents for seeking professional mental health counseling after the loss of a child, but when stressors seem more mundane and ordinary, there is often a failure to recognize the impact.

Major incidences leave permanent scars on a person's psyche. That permanent mark on the brain circuitry must be dealt with or else the battles will last a lifetime. Resilience is powerful, but it cannot always put all the broken pieces back together.

It should be starting to become obvious: fear takes many forms and has many faces. Fear is defined differently for everyone, and we all have different fears and those fears affect us in a variety of ways.

If we do not deal with our fears and try ignoring them, our fear becomes like a quicksand from which you cannot emerge. And like quicksand, the more you fight it, the worse it gets. Through a process called *potentiation*, the fear response is increasingly amplified. In the medical world, the combination of two drugs might produce a better result than simply using one or the other alone. In the example of fear, however, potentiation—combining one fear with another (and perhaps another)—is never going to be positive.

When a person is already primed for fear, events, even those that are essentially harmless, seem frightening. Everyone has watched a documentary about spiders or bugs only to jump hysterically when a sweater thread tickles the skin on the back of the neck. People who are nervous about flying panic at the slightest turbulence mid-flight.

To understand our fears better, consider why people become afraid in the first place. Fear is a natural reaction essential for human survival. Fear helps form the basic fight-or-flight response that gives people the courage needed to take a defensive stance or a warning system to escape danger. A simple yet accurate definition of fear is an anxious feeling that can be induced by the anticipation of an event. The body responds to fears in almost the exact same way no matter what the source of the fear might be.

Dr. Karl Albrecht, developer of the hierarchy of fear titled "feararchy," posits all fears come from one of five categories. By breaking fears down into these categories, it becomes easier to see what it is people *truly* fear: extinction, mutilation, loss of autonomy, separation, and ego death.

It should be no shock that **extinction** is at the top of Albrecht's list.

The fear of dying, of ceasing to exist, is what prompts humans to fight for survival. The idea of no longer *being* strikes at the very heart of the human condition. The fear of extinction, however, is not merely the fear of dying. It is also the fear of doing something that could lead to death. The racing heart and the fast-paced breaths following a near miss on the freeway stems from the fear of extinction. And while everyone has near misses or panicked moments when calamity is avoided, the fear of extinction can be life-controlling in some people.

For example, a person with a severe fear of heights is basically suffering from a fear of extinction. It is not so much that he is afraid of looking off a high cliff or from the top floor of a skyscraper. Rather, he is afraid of the imagined extinction that could befall him should he lose footing, slip, and tumble to his death.

Second on Albrecht's list is the fear of **mutilation**. It is the idea that some part of our body could be destroyed or rendered unusable. As always, some fears are founded in logic. A person who has been diagnosed with macular degeneration might have a legitimate fear of eventually losing her eyesight. However, most people have no real reason to fear blindness. Likewise, fears of feeling unsafe in particular situations would fall into the category of fear of mutilation. The fear of mutilation is the root of many common fears, no matter how irrational they may seem.

A person afraid of animals like dogs or snakes is really not afraid of the creature; they fear the potential mutilation the creature could impose. Fear of needles, going to the dentist, or getting lost in a crowd are really fears about what could happen when something goes wrong in that particular situation. Dentists are not frightening in and of themselves, but when imagining the mutilation, which could include the potential for inflicted pain, some people become petrified.

Albrecht's third basic fear is the fear of **loss of autonomy**—in other words, loss of control.

Loss of autonomy is most often associated with loss of physical control, though not always—in other words, when a person is restricted in some way and cannot move, cannot breathe, is trapped, is imprisoned, or is paralyzed. Most people are familiar with the term claustrophobia and can have some sort of paralyzing fear of being caught and unable to escape.

Loss of autonomy can go beyond the feeling of claustrophobia in an elevator for three hours. It can also have serious repercussions on our relationships. It is not uncommon for couples to feel trapped in an unhappy marriage because they see no way out;

employees can feel ensnared in an unsatisfactory job because of financial burdens; elderly people feel confined because of the physical limitations that keep them from the freedoms they once took for granted; even parents can feel stuck with the responsibilities of raising children with no vision of living for themselves on the horizon.

And what happens when we feel a loss of freedom and autonomy? We desperately want it back. At its most extreme, people can feel caught in a web of hopelessness and feel there is no way out without ending it all.

The fear of **separation, abandonment, and rejection** haunts the human condition. The previous fear categories were mostly physical by nature; now we turn to what we want to avoid psychologically.

One of the first emotions infants experience is separation and abandonment. Research and common sense tells us that a baby who cries and then is comforted with the human touch learns to trust, while babies who are neglected fail to thrive. That desire to be connected to others never ceases. Everyone seeks to be accepted, and those who are not constantly struggle with the fear of being rejected.

While there are certainly many triggers that can increase the fear of separation and abandonment within a person, some obvious ones include the end of a friendship, death, loss, or divorce. In order to avoid this fear, some people will go the extreme to avoid any real types of intimacy.

Thoughts including things like "If I do not make myself vulnerable, then I will not get hurt" or "If I do not care about the relationship, then if it ends then I will not feel heartbroken" allow a person to convince himself intimacy is not worth the effort. And while avoiding close relationships does eliminate arguments and disagreements and could be a good coping mechanism for a marble statue, humans need real relationships that require each person to invest in the other.

For many people, being rejected is their greatest fear. This is really what comes up the most in their lives. It comes to mean "I am not worthy" or "I am not good enough as a human being." If can also cause people to try to compensate in hopes of making others see their value. "Perhaps if I behave properly he will love me" or "Maybe if I lose 50 pounds someone with think I am beautiful or If I could just earn this degree they will be proud of me."

And while most people deal with the fear of being rejected by individuals, a friend, a spouse, a parent, a lover, there is also a strong fear of being rejected by a group or society at large. Being on the outs with the mean girls in middle school can be painfully difficult, and being disowned by family members can bring a lifetime of hurt. Evolutionarily speaking, being rejected from society as a whole can be life-threatening. According to Albrecht, separation, abandonment, and rejection can lead to a "loss of connectedness; of becoming a non-person—not wanted, respected, or valued by anyone else." This can literally threaten our well-being and survival.

Finally, Albrecht offers the fear of **ego death or humiliation.** How can we possibly forget Marcia Brady and her imagining the entire school sitting in their underwear before giving her big speech? Why did she get that advice? Because she was nervous about humiliating herself in front of the whole school. And just like *Marcia, Marcia, Marcia*, the number one fear people have is public speaking.

No one likes being made to feel ashamed. Even a puppy will lower its head and slink around after making an accident on the carpet. Shame can make people feel worthless, and most people will go to great lengths to avoid that. Misspeaking in a presentation, falling up the stairs, or completing an entire conversation with spinach between two teeth can be mortifying. It can make people feel humiliated, unworthy, and unlovable at worst and unprepared, silly, and embarrassed at best.

There are many things that can cause shame, and some are certainly more serious than others. Like fear, shame can be a good thing. For example, a person should feel guilt or shame when telling a lie or working a dishonest business deal. However, people most often feel shame over things they cannot control, like a lost job or a stolen briefcase. Even more troublesome is when someone feels shame after being victimized. Shame can certainly become debilitating in certain situations.

Albrecht's feararchy is helpful in naming and identifying the most common ways we hold ourselves back. Do you see yourself reflected in any of the categories? Perhaps all of them? Whatever the case, it's imperative to put a label on what you're dealing with so you can fight it with the right approach.

The intention of this book is to give readers the necessary tools to remove fear in their lives—to cut it out, to perform the formidoectomy, and to end the control it has on them. Know that fear only has the power to keep you where you are if you give it that power. Armed with knowledge about your fears, tools to overcome your fears, and an action plan to eliminate your fears once and for all, you will be able to move closer to the person you want to be.

Takeaways:

- Fear is not something we can control, even though it is one of the most basic human feelings. Fear may have had purposes in the past, but it seems like it only serves to keep us from what we desire these days.
- We fear *fear* more than anything else, and sometimes this is because we feel a lack of control. We may not always fear the actual consequences, but the uncertainty can be paralyzing. Therefore, it is best to stop fixating and creating an imagined nightmare in your head and focus on what is possible to control.
- Though we are all familiar with traumatic experiences and the toll they can have, sometimes we ignore how stress and anxiety can build up from daily reactions

to fear. They are just as important to deal with and shouldn't be overlooked.

- Dr. Karl Albrecht developed what he called a feararchy, which documented the five most prevalent and universal fears. They include extinction, mutilation, loss of autonomy, separation and rejection, and humiliation.

Chapter 2. The Origins of Fear

This chapter discusses the evolutionary and biological origins of fear. As with many aspects of our daily existence, fear exists for a reason. In our ancestral past, fear was a major factor that allowed our species to flourish. Even in today's modern world, without the threat of saber-toothed tigers and other species that viewed us as food, fear plays an important role in keeping people safe and, in some cases, alive.

Fear itself is not bad. What makes fear bad is how individuals react to it.

In reality, fear is neutral. It is a biological signal, similar to the stimulations of hot and cold. When a person feels extreme heat, the nerve cells send a message to the brain and the brain interprets the signal and directs the body to pull away. If all works correctly, the biological signal saves the person from a burn. Likewise, fear is a signal being sent to the brain. The brain must interpret the signal and then direct the body to take an action.

And this is wherein the problem lies. The fear signal gets sent, but for the most part, the brain, despite best intentions, does not interpret fear to be useful or positive.

This is because fear signals the *freeze, fight, flight, or fright* response in humans (Steimer, 2002). Everyone has experienced this response first hand and seen it in action in nature. On a hike in the woods, a snapped twig will cause a doe and her baby to make direct eye contact with a human. This last a split second before the doe instinctively knows running to escape the perceived danger will protect both herself and her young.

Like the doe, humans have a mechanism that tells us to freeze. Whether we are walking the crowded streets at rush hour or approaching an unfriendly dog, fear is the trigger that says *Stop. Look. Listen.* Fear is our signal to pay close attention, put the senses on high alert, and react appropriately.

At times, that warning is needed. But on a daily basis, people must develop a sense of discrimination in order to understand when the triggered fear is necessary and helpful versus when it is unhelpful and only hindering daily living. Of course, this is how post-traumatic stress disorder (PTSD) functions— victims are unable to stop perceiving everything as a true threat, so their fear and anxiety systems are perpetually engaged.

Many of us engage in this theater as well, albeit unknowingly because of the biological means we process fear.

Humans respond to a fearful stimulus through a process of three steps: freeze, fight or flight, and fright (Bracha, 2004). Through millennia of evolution this has kept the species alive. The key is to calibrate the response appropriately. Looking at each response, it is easy to see how people can make healthy, rational decisions about the thing they fear or completely irrational ones.

The first response is **freeze**. It simply means that the person stops what he or she is doing to focus on the fearful stimulus and consider the best course of action. An employee reads a memo stating there will layoffs at the end of the year; she stops to consider what that could mean for her. A car horn blasts as a person steps off a curb; he stops and considers the safest option.

Sometimes the freeze lasts just a few seconds. Consider the person on the curb, who better react instantly to preserve his own life, but sometimes some processing time is required. It is during this freeze time that a plan about what to do next begins to take shape. Sometimes this response is altogether skipped if there is a large enough fear.

The next response is going to be one of two options: either **fight or flight**. Back to the nature walk scenario, the doe, in an effort to protect herself and her fawn, will run. If, however, the nature walk includes a flock of geese and their babies, there will be no animals running off to hide. The mother goose will charge a human, beating her wings wildly and squawking to wake the dead. The doe will always choose flight; the goose will always choose fight.

Unlike geese, humans do not get an automatic, preprogrammed response to fearful situations. And while sometimes the choice is more obvious than it is at other times, it is always necessary to make some sort of decision.

Back to the email stating there will be layoffs at the end of the year. The employee on the receiving end of that message must decide the best option: fight or flight. Fighting would include having conversations with the boss about her performance, her role as a valuable asset to the company, or the possibility of additional responsibilities that improve her position within the company.

Her flight response would be to start looking for another job, updating her résumé, networking with colleagues in her field, or considering options of breaking out on her own. Fight is not a bad option; flight is not a bad option. After receiving the initial fear-inducing stimulus, freezing to consider the options and then making decisions about what the next step should be are rational steps for dealing with a fear-provoking situation.

A more common example might simply be seeing an intimidating person walk toward you in a dark alley. Your heart will start pounding and you may begin to shake from the release of adrenaline into your system. When the mystery man gets closer and closer, you will feel compelled to choose between standing your ground and fighting or turning and sprinting away as fast as you can. Whatever the case, your body is ready.

The final response to a fear-inducing stimulus is **fright**. When the fear is overwhelming to the point that the person can neither fight nor flee, then fright takes over. Rather than considering options, making a plan, or taking action, the person is stuck obsessing, ruminating, complaining, yet doing nothing to change the situation. Being continuously in fright mode can lead to hopelessness and depression. Fright is a lack of action yet continued stress and anxiety. Of course, that's if you let yourself perceive fear in that way.

The Biology of Fear

To gain a full understanding of fear as a natural occurrence, it is important to understand the biology behind it. Fear is hardwired into everyone's brain for a good reason.

Neuroscientists have identified distinct networks that run from the depths of the limbic system all the way to prefrontal cortex of the brain and back. When a person experiences a fear-inducing stimulus, this part of the brain kicks into action and causes him to experience fear. Interestingly, when these networks are electronically or chemically stimulated, they also produce fear, even in the complete absence of a naturally fearful stimulus.

Feeling fear is a natural part of being human. It is not abnormal, nor is it a sign of weakness. In fact, the ability to experience fear is a perfectly normal aspect of brain function. The lack of fear may actually be a sign of serious brain damage.

When a person feels fear, there are two primary pathways within the brain fear can take.

One path is subconscious, implicit, and almost instantaneous. This is the primary pathway. The other path is conscious, explicit, and much, much slower. Of course, this is the secondary pathway.

The primary pathway is associated with the amygdala within the brain. When a person senses danger, the amygdala takes over and instantly discharges patterns to activate the body's fear circuits. This causes an increase in heart rate and blood pressure. Additional physiological responses include sweaty hands, dry mouth, and tense muscles.

This is the perfect response in many dangerous situations because it prepares the body to respond to a threat by either standing up to it or running away from it (fight or flight). When the blood flow is diverted quickly from the digestive area, the face, head, and neck, then it can be used elsewhere. And while a fist fight or a sprint from the situation is not often necessary in this modern world, the brain and body prepare just for those possible reactions. This is the reason people experience a racing heart and shortness of breath after being frightened.

The secondary and explicit pathway is the more thoughtful way we deal with a fearful stimulus.

Rather than being directed by the amygdala, this response is directed by the hippocampus, which is the structure within the brain that supports explicit or conscious memory. The hippocampus also provides context for the human experience. For example, it is the hippocampus that allows people to learn about and assess their surroundings in order to determine the levels of threat or friendliness. Additionally, the hippocampus is particularly sensitive to encoding the context associated with an aversive or painful experience.

The hippocampus is particularly active when people experience trauma within relationships. It only takes a small amount of fear stimulus for the hippocampus to condition a person to associate a particular stimulus with a conditioned fear. Additionally, objects and/or locations associated with the fear can also become a source of conditioned fear. This is how painful memories from old relationships can become generalized or projected into new ones.

An example of the hippocampus at work can be seen perpetuating the cycle of fear within families where shouting and yelling were predominant forms of punishment. A young girl comes to associate persistent screaming, racket, and hollering with family pain and chaos. As an adult, when her boyfriend or husband yells at her, she associates that ruckus with the family pain she experienced as a child. Therefore, when an argument starts and he raises his voice, her response is much like it was as a child: fight, run, or remain stuck in fright.

The primary response is automatic and happens with little thought, and this causes us to leap *before* we look. The secondary response that runs through the hippocampus is slower and can range from seconds to minutes of processing. Unlike the child whose upbringing is surrounded by constant shouting and screaming, a child who is yelled at for darting into the street without looking both ways is not going to associate raised voices with chaos and family pain that eventually leads to a fright response when her husband speaks loudly to her. The purpose of this book is to teach readers to deal with both types of responses to fear.

Fear also produces physiological changes, a few of which we have mentioned. When a person perceives a fear stimulus, adrenaline prepares the skeletal muscles to deal with whatever decision is made—fight or flight. As stated above, blood flow moves toward those essential body parts need to run away or pull the fists and fight it out. However, there can be complications associated with these reactions.

First, if the blood flows away from the brain too quickly, then there a several possible reactions, none of which help with the fight-or-flight response. A person could faint, feel numbness, or freeze. At the most basic human survival level, this reaction is unlikely to end with a positive result. Even in our modern society, however, fainting during a stressful event, feeling numb and unsure of a response when given shocking news, or freezing up before making an important announcement are not conducive to reducing fears.

Second, when the body produces adrenaline in preparation for a physical fight-or-flight response, and then there is no vigorous physical activity after that arousal, uncomfortable physiological changes can occur. For example, many people experience sensations including trembling in their arms or legs, general weakness, or a heightened awareness of breathing and heart rate. If the adrenaline goes unused, imagine how you might feel after having four cups of coffee.

What if that happens time after time and a person cannot flee (run away) or fight (face the fear stimulus)? Those biological urges can become hardwired and habitual. Physically, the body has prepared to do something drastic, but what happens if those intentions or actions are never taken? These urges to flee or fight, these actions that were never taken, can get triggered repeatedly, especially when old, unresolved fear and hurt from the past are triggered by relationships in the present.

These can emerge as transference reactions or projections onto others. Furthermore, they could drive reenactment patterns that cause people to repeat the same mistakes in relationship after relationship in spite of their desire and commitment to avoid such blunders.

The biology of fear seems destined to only affect us in negative ways, but the truth is, we needed to have intense fear reactions to stay alive for most of human history. We are now in the business of deprogramming our brains of instinct, which is even more deeply ingrained than habit. It's a difficult but necessary road.

The Origins of Fear

Understanding that fear starts as a biological response to a stimulus, we can explore why we are afraid of certain things. Where does fear originate?

Certainly, major parts of it are through instinct, but there are also *learned* and *taught* aspects. Instinctual fears are those things that are feared in order to ensure survival. From the beginning of time, mankind has feared large beasts because of the threat they pose to survival. In the modern world, people might fear dirty looking food because they are worried about contracting a particular disease or disorder.

Some instinctual fears are rational, while others seem to have little basis in reality. For example, a fear of sharks is not irrational when vacationing at the beach and "Beware of the Sharks" signs are posted at regular intervals. Sitting in the Midwest, thousands of miles from salt water, however, seems like an unreasonable place feel petrified of a shark attack.

In spite of the fact that these instinctual fears can morph into something irrational, biologically, people are designed to fear these things. It is not irrational to have an innate fear of sharks, snakes, wild boars, people with guns, tornadoes, and speeding semi-trucks. We are genetically predisposed to fear things with the potential to harm (Tsaousides, 2015).

Other fears are learned. Being afraid of certain people, places, or situations is caused because of negative associations and past experiences. A common learned fear has to do with water. A near-drowning experience can cause a person to be afraid of getting close to water or even watching others in the water—especially people they care about. Similarly, surviving a dangerous car wreck can cause people to be fearful of driving at high speeds or over bridges.

Like instinctual fears, learned fears, while acquired through learning and conditioning, are quite normal fears. Having an experience with a scary result is a natural reason for developing a fear.

Finally, there are fears that are taught. It could be that a mother who survived a near-drowning experience teaches her children to fear the water; however, many taught fears are far more sinister. Oftentimes, cultural norms dictate whether or not something should be feared. Racism is a classic example of how one social group assigns negative character traits to another social group, and the eventual result is that both groups fear each other. In its extreme, this can lead to persecution, imprisonment, and genocide.

A final source of fear is the ever-vivid imagination, and it is present in instinctual, learned, and taught fears.

While imagination is *sometimes* rooted in an actual fear, people often allow their brains to convince them something is scary even when it is not. A person who is afraid of snakes may have a legitimate instinctual fear of being bitten by a snake or could even have an actual learned fear after being bitten by a snake. It makes sense that this person would have a fearful reaction to seeing a snake, real or fake, that would look like fear. The psychological term for this is *conditioned fear*. However, when there is no snake around, no books about snakes, no television commercials with snakes, or no toy snakes on the coffee table, the person could still struggle with extremely fearful reactions because of what is called *anticipatory anxiety*.

Some neuroscientists claim humans are the most fearful creatures on the planet. This is not because of our inability to defend ourselves from scary things, but rather because of our ability to learn, think, and create fear in our minds. Humans have the unique ability to take a low-grade, objectless fear and turn it into chronic anxiety. This anxiety, this worry about that which only exists within the imagination, can become debilitating.

When Fear Is Your Friend

While the focus of this book is assisting you with overcoming fear and learning to live a courageous and fulfilling life, it is essential to recognize that fear has many helpful roles in life. Without a healthy sense of fear, humans would not have made it to this point on the evolutionary trail. Even in this modern age, fear can be our lighthouse in the dark seas.

Fear serves as a **protector.** You know this already. When a person is afraid of something, it is often for good reason. What they fear could have both the power and the potential to bring harm. When the brain identifies a threat, the hypothalamus is triggered, thus letting the rest of the body know how best to prepare for whatever might be coming.

Afterward, the adrenal glands release adrenaline to alert the nervous system that it is time to get into survival mode (either fight or flight). Another hormone, norepinephrine, is also released during this period. Its purpose is to improve focus while reducing panic. Jake Deutsch, MD, an emergency room physician, says norepinephrine "allows clearer thinking under stress, which is precisely why it's used in many antidepressants." Thus, being in a panicky situation is far more likely to help someone think quickly and clearly than chugging another energy drink or reaching for a triple espresso latte.

Who can forget the Miracle on the Hudson? In 2009, Captain Chesley B. Sullivan landed a plane filled with 155 passengers and crew in the middle of the Hudson River in New York City after birds damaged the engines. With all those lives in his hands, "Sully" was able to remain calm under extreme pressure and land safely. His ability to focus all of his energy into saving that plane prevented a terrible disaster.

Fear serves as a **motivator**. University certainly brings out the "fear as motivator" theme like few other life experiences. At one time, in the not so distant past, it meant sliding the final paper into the assignment slot in the English Department office before 8:00 a.m. on the last day of class. Now students upload the drafts to the portal by 11:59 p.m. or hit send just as the deadline approaches. The technology may have changed, but students have not. And nothing lights the motivational fires like the looming deadline of semester's end.

It is not just on campus, however, that fear motivates. There's this old joke. The new guy asks his mentor, "How long have you worked here?" The mentor answers, "I've been here 10 years, but I started working last month when they threatened to fire me." And while it is a knee-slapper at motivational conventions worldwide, there is a lot of truth in it. Fear can be an incredible motivator, especially when trying to accomplish career and workplace goals.

Debbie Mandel, stress-management specialist and the author of *Addicted to Stress*, says an adrenaline rush not only helps you delegate and become a productive team member, but it also is needed by many during the "eleventh hour, whether it's to tackle a project at work or write a paper on a deadline."

Finally, fear is your **analyst**. Fear does not show up in life without reason. Typically, there is a fear that needs tackling, and the only way to do so is to face it head on. If you're experiencing fear, it does you good to ask what is causing it and for what purpose. In life, thoughts of failure or loss naturally cause people to do everything possible to avoid those experiences.

Sometimes the only way to avoid becoming a victim of a fear is to analyze the fear. Asking questions like "What am I actually afraid of?" and "What can I do to overcome this fear?" allows people to work through the obstacles that hold them back while looking for new ways to take proactive steps in a new direction.

In order to help answer these difficult questions, the focus on the next chapter will be the real and tangible types of fears we face in our everyday lives—the ones that people feel hold them back and keep them from realizing their fullest potential. As we move ahead, try to identify your fears. Consider the things you would like to do but you feel like you can't because of fear. Know that as you move through this book, you will be able to not only identify them, but also overcome them.

Takeaways:

- Even though it seems that fear's only purpose is to keep us from what we want in life, fear has been one of the most powerful safeguards to life. This is because of how we respond to a fear stimulus: *freeze, fight, flight, or fright.* Biologically speaking, that is how your brain will process fear and cause you to act. Thus, much of what we want to accomplish in this book is to go against your ingrained instincts.

- There are two main pathways for fear: a primary and secondary pathway. The primary pathway is instantaneous and subconscious, and it is what triggers the three-step fear response. The secondary pathway is slower and conscious, and it causes us to ask, "What is the problem here and how do I deal with it?"
- Fears are mostly instinctual, but they can also be learned and taught. These are no easier to shed.
- Despite the negatives of fear, it still has three important roles in our lives. If you care to listen and not react by fighting or fleeing, fear can act as your protector, motivator, and analyst.

Chapter 3. What Really Matters

At the end of Chapter 1, there was a discussion about Albrecht's five types of fear. When considering the fears people face, it can be helpful to categorize them into one of those five basic fears.

His categorization, however, is more theoretical in nature. In real day-to-day life, most people do not consider how to classify their fears. Even though everyone has fears concerning physical harm, few pick up books like this one to help them overcome their fear of getting mutilated or maimed. That's just not what fear means to us in a tangible sense.

Most readers are hoping to figure out how to gain control of the fears that hold them back in social situations—whether that is related to their careers, family, or personal relationships. Perhaps your fear is that you are never going to find someone with whom you can share life.

Or perhaps you are worried that you are never going to mend the broken relationship you have with a dear friend. Instead of worrying about the way the things are compared to the way you want them to be, identify them for what they are. Soon you will have a clear strategy to make the changes you so desperately want.

Fear of Failure

The greatest fear most of us face is the fear of failure—which includes rejection. Often, the words *failure* and *rejection* are used interchangeably because the fear is essentially the same.

Typically, the term *rejection* is used to describe fear associated with people, while *failure* is most often associated with feelings of feeling inadequate by falling short or failing to measure up to expectations in some way. Over time, fear of failure can become paralyzing. It can cause people to reach a point where the only thing they can do is nothing at all. It rarely happens all at once. A single failure or two is not going to cause a person to give up completely, but gradually, if a person tries and tries without hints of success, a person could eventually reach a point where, unless there is a nearly 100% guaranteed success rate, there is little motivation to try.

This can be as innocent as not trying out for the basketball team in case you don't make it, and it can be as detrimental as never applying for jobs because you don't want to experience the feeling of rejection.

This phenomenon is known in the scientific community as *learned helplessness*. Psychologists Martin Seligman and Steve Maier discovered during a series of experiments that dogs who had previously "learned" that their efforts didn't prevent shocks simply adopted the mindset of whining and giving up even when placed in situations where they could easily have escaped a shock.

Unlike the dogs in the experiment, humans rarely lie down and accept an electric shock; however, it is not uncommon for people to view their actions as having no effect on the situation, even when those actions could result in avoiding something negative or unpleasant. The individual loses hope and believes the situation is beyond control; therefore, the response is to accept the situation. Like the dogs in the experiment, when people experience a strong blow of rejection, the best reaction seems to be to lie down and whine.

When people do nothing at all, they do not get the chance to fail or be rejected. For many, that seems like the best option. People would rather remain blissfully ignorant instead of confirming a negative self-identity, lack of ability, or inadequacy. Therefore, they will avoid taking any action that could change the status quo.

In other words, fear of failure, which includes fear of rejection and fear of inadequacy, comes down to this: people are afraid of not being good enough. This can be paralyzing. It often feels safer to keep goals a secret and avoid pursuing new dreams because then there is no chance of discovering *I am not good enough.* Imagine the thing people miss because they are not willing to risk failure— the fun, the adventure, the joy. When people focus on avoiding failure, worrying about failure becomes the focus rather than the effort needed to reach goals.

Learned helplessness can even show up in relationships. Parents are often guilty of creating a sense of learned helplessness within their children. Recall the painstaking patience required when teaching a child to tie his shoe. Even though it is a milestone accomplishment, it can take weeks or months before a child can tie his shoes quickly. Nagging, scolding, and huffy breathing do nothing to help increase his pace. In the midst of the morning rush, the ball practice rush, or the playdate rush, it really is easier (and faster) to simply tie the kid's shoes and get moving.

And while shoe-tying seems like such a small thing, children can become victims of learned helplessness quickly: "When something is hard, eventually Mom or Dad will do it for me." If parents are not careful, it stops being about tying shoes and starts being about anything that does not come naturally with little effort or practice. It's a mindset that can last through adulthood: "I can't do anything about it, so forget it."

Humans are extremely sensitive to rejection, especially forms of *social* rejection. Most people have strong motivation to seek approval and acceptance. From the start of human history, humans have had the need for social relationships. Taking an anthropological perspective, the reason people lived in tribal communities was for survival. Ten thousand years ago, a person could not survive alone. Tribes provided food, shelter, and protection. Being rejected by the tribe was the ultimate punishment because it meant imminent death. Evolutionarily speaking, humans are hardwired to form social relationships and are strongly motivated to feel accepted.

Everyone has felt the sting of rejection at some point in life. Interestingly, MRI studies show the same areas of the brain are activated when a person experiences rejection as when a person experiences physical pain. Neurologically speaking, rejection can hurt just as much as a broken bone or twisted ankle. Therefore, people, in an effort to avoid the pain of rejection, may choose to isolate themselves from others to avoid pain.

One of the best ways of overcoming a fear of failing is having a lot of practice failing. It's not necessarily that you should strive to fail, but rather that it is possible to become immunized to how it feels. Once you fail and realize that the world hasn't ended and nothing much has changed except for the fact that you need to start over, failure becomes less daunting and merely annoying. You change the association from massive pain to frustration at having to persevere.

Aside from getting a lot of practice failing, another way to overcome fear is to embrace failure as a learning experience. If failure is one of life's greatest teachers, then it is wasted on us if we do not learn something from it. Thomas Edison has been cited for discovering over 1000 ways *not* to make a light bulb. Perhaps you have learned how *not* to do something, but you have stopped trying to learn *how* to do it. Let your failed attempts teach you so you can do better next time.

Fear of Judgment

Second only to the fear of failure is the fear of being judged by others. This is another social fear. Simply put, humans are afraid of what other people might think about them. Those who are self-conscious are afraid others will think they are stupid, incapable, or inadequate. No surprise, the fear of being judged keeps people from trying new things.

People will go to self-defeating lengths to elude the possibility of being negatively judged by others. They avoid having difficult conversations, even when they have something to say that is critical to the relationship. They do not speak up in class or at work meetings; they avoid telling their lover their true desires; they will not ask for a raise; they answer "I don't care" when asked by a date where to have dinner.

This fear of judgment is linked to an inner desire to be liked by all at all times. How is that even possible? And yet according to Watson and Friend's research in 1969, this desire, compounded by low self-worth and self-esteem, keeps people from uninhibitedly experiencing and expressing their true selves.

Judgment is unavoidable. Everyone makes judgments concerning others every day. No one can control what others think; what people can do, however, is help others understand the context of feelings. By being open and honest, people give others the chance to show compassion. And compassion is judgment's kryptonite. When compassion is present, judgments have very little weight because people can imagine themselves feeling the same way.

Consider this: the human brain has limited data reserves. Although judgments are made regularly, they are often not significant enough to earn a place in the memory bank for eternity. Therefore, when someone makes a judgment, chances are that in just a few moments, or at most a few days, that judgment will have left their conscious awareness. People develop an understanding of others based on patterns of behaviors and lasting impressions over time rather than on minor mistakes or temporary setbacks. It may feel differently, but we are not the center of people's attention.

Individuals often live life feeling like they are in the spotlight, but generally that simply is not true. A misstep on the stairs or bit of spittle when speaking might feel magnified for the whole room to see, but the reality is, most people either did not see it or did not notice it enough for the event to register and make a lasting impression. Judgment can be scary when it confirms our worst beliefs, but most of the time, people don't care enough to judge.

One of the most practical steps to take in overcoming a fear of judgment is to realize only the famous people are constantly being watched. Normal, everyday people are generally ignored by most people most of the time. Media, a 24-hour news cycle, and the paparazzi have given us a skewed view of what people look at in everyday, normal life.

Obviously, everyone has moments in the spotlight—for example, when speaking up during a discussion or making a presentation—but even then, all eyes and all attention is not 100% focused during that period of time. Additionally, by recognizing that self-criticism is much harsher than any other criticism, it becomes possible to move past blunders.

Another helpful step in overcoming a fear of judgment is to stop letting the opinion of others play such an important role in defining self-worth.

Admitting that people are regularly passing some sort of judgment, yet recognizing that their opinion really does not matter in terms of personal success or value, is an essential step. Instead of focusing on the opinions of others, focus on what you like about yourself and what you're good at. Admittedly, that could take some hard work, and perhaps even some professional help, but discovering self-worth outside of another's view is a fundamental element of confidence.

Finally, a fear of being judged often keeps people from trying new things or pushing their own limits. There is a very real cost-benefit to weigh—what are you missing out on because you care what others might think of you? When you perform this mental calculus, you might realize that you are being held back by a *split second* of fear from something that could provide you with years or enjoyment or happiness. It's frequent that we are avoiding something small that happens to be a gatekeeper to what we really want in life.

For example, a person may avoid starting a 5K training program because she fears confirming her suspicions that she is not an athlete. Yet when she realizes all her friends and family run, as do many eligible single men, she'll find that she is missing out on all of that—and for what, exactly? Not much.

Fear of Change and the Unknown

"If nothing ever changed, there would be no butterflies." While the originator of that aphorism is unknown, the profound wisdom can help people see the necessity of change. And yet, so many people live in constant fear of change.

Just like fear itself, change is neutral and only depends on interpretation. Change can be seen as positive, like moving to a new home or starting a new job, or it can be seen as negative like the death of a loved one or a divorce. Any event that requires an adjustment in day-to-day life, even when it is positive, can cause stress and fear.

One reason people fear change is because they live life thinking "This just might be as good as it gets." This mindset causes people to settle for the status quo rather than taking a risk. While going back to school to add a degree or certification could result in a promotion or better job, it will bring change to everyday life. Therefore, some people would prefer to remain stuck where they are instead of upsetting the proverbial apple cart.

Similarly, people fear that change might leave them in a worse position than before. Going back to school may have its benefits, but there are no guarantees. There will be tuition costs, time costs, and childcare costs, but there is no promise that the promotion or better job will come. Therefore, someone could talk himself out of returning to school because of the fear he would be in a worse position than before. Instead of thinking "This might be as good as it gets," he thinks "This could end up being a whole lot worse."

In Chapter 1 there was a discussion about how fear makes people feel out of control. Change also makes people feel out of control, and when a person is out of control, he or she becomes fearful. Uncertainty is a part of life. Everyone has to accept that, and obviously sooner is better than later.

Sometimes change happens because of personal choice. A decision to take a job on the other side of the world is exciting and full of possibilities. Yet, it is full of unknowns. Questions like "Where will I live? Will I make enough money to meet my needs? Do I need a car? Will I make friends? What if there is an emergency and I need to come home?" snowball with hundreds more legitimate concerns when considering an international move. And yet, people do it all the time. Even under the best circumstances, there can still be apprehension.

Sometimes change happens because of circumstances that are completely uncontrollable. The death of a spouse is a prime example. Suddenly, one person who has been part of a team is left alone to manage everything—kids, home, finances, and family. The responsibilities of being a surviving spouse are enormous but really nothing compared to the grief. In a situation like this, fear seems like a fairly reasonable response.

Like overcoming any other fear, overcoming the fear of change and the unknown is not easy. If the change is not by choice, then it can be especially difficult to get over the fears.

Attempt to avoid focusing on everything that could go wrong. It would be a statistical impossibility for everything to go exactly to plan during times of change, but that certainly does not equate failure. It just means that planning is never perfect, and life has a way of being unpredictable. Focusing on the possibility of failure results in ignoring the endless possibilities of things going right—probably in unexpected and unimaginable ways. While complete, utter, and total failure is conceivable, it is just one tiny possibility in a sea of unknown outcomes.

When change is occurring by choice, it is because the individual knows a change is what she needs. There is something out there better for her than what she has now. The only way for her to get it is to incite the change. This is the time to get excited and embrace the idea of discovering all the possibilities, finding a better life, and being happier. The future may seem exhilarating, but the key is to conquer the fear. Allowing fear to be the reigning emotion, as opposed to excitement, anticipation, or expectation, robs people of the joy of becoming their best self.

Finally, when change seems intimidating, it can be helpful to focus on the things in your life that remain unfaltering and unchanged. Things that cannot be taken away can become like an anchor that holds steadfast even in the most frightening situations. Even in a whirlwind of unknown possibilities, some things will not change: certain strong relationships, personal resolve, creative talents, and faith. Holding on to these constants can be helpful during times of change and anchor you to reality and positivity.

Fear of Success

Some readers are thinking "How can this be a thing? Who doesn't want success?" It is, however, a real fear that many people have, even if they cannot articulate it. We all have known people who seem to sabotage nearly every chance at success they have. The reasons for fearing success are as varied as the people who have the fear.

Some people fear success because they fear having the spotlight on themselves. Recall that people who fear judgment feel like they are always in the spotlight, always being watched, always being judged. The more attention, the more naysayers that will come out of the woods. This can be especially problematic when others start pointing out faults or finding ways to second-guess decisions.

When someone is successful, others often put that person on a pedestal, seek advice, or try to emulate his behavior. That can feel like a lot of pressure, a lot of unwanted pressure. For someone who does not like pressure, that can become overwhelming. He may not feel like he can cope with it.

Another reason people fear success is because they fear it leaving after a period of time, and they are afraid of their inability to cope. Everyone has heard stories of lottery winners who are broke a mere five years after becoming millionaires. People do not like to have something and then lose it. The idea of achieving success, whatever that looks like, and indulging in the spoils of success, whatever those may be—wealth, fame, relationships—and then losing it all, feels like a lot to risk. Some people seem to create a self-fulfilling prophecy of failure in order avoid the responsibility that comes with success.

Oftentimes success comes via change. After all, if you keep doing what you've been doing, there's no reason to expect to get a bigger reward.

Perhaps a change in education level led to a new job. Perhaps a new business idea took off at just the right time. Perhaps an unexpected connection quickly turned into a relationship. If a person struggles with a fear of change, then it is likely they would also struggle if that change brought about success. It seems like an odd dichotomy—that one could be fearful of both change and the success that might come with it. Many people, however, are comfortable with things just the way they are.

Finally, people fear success because they are afraid they might be discovered for who they really are. This is *imposter syndrome*. Remember the movie *Catch Me If You Can*. Leonardo di Caprio played the character based on the real person Frank Abagnale, who was indeed a fraud. He created credentials and impersonated airline pilots, doctors, and millionaires, but he was really nothing more than gutsy kid with a mature-looking face and good hand for forging checks.

Obviously, there are very few Frank Abagnales in the world, but there are certainly people who feel like they are in over their heads and that, someday, someone is going to find out they are a fraud. Perhaps it is the graduate student who is teaching two sections of freshman composition who feels like she is barely qualified to take courses, let alone teach them.

Perhaps it is the manager who dreads the day he has to settle a dispute between two employees because he hates conflict. Perhaps it is the founder's daughter who has to step in and run the family business after her father's death. It is not so much that they really are frauds, but they feel that they are in a position for which they are grossly underqualified.

Just like some other fears mentioned in this chapter, working on improving self-esteem and confidence can help people become calmer about success. Focusing on your positive traits and your strengths can help build your confidence. Do not be afraid to highlight your best traits either. Are you a really good listener? Then use that skill as you try to build relationships. Are you super organized? Make sure that is apparent in all the work you do.

A final way to avoid fearing success comes in the old adage *fake it till you make it*. We have all been in situations where we felt like we were in over our heads. And while it may feel a bit disingenuous at first, sometimes there is no other way to go except along like you belong.

If the graduate student starts to view herself as a scholar and a teacher, she will start to feel like she belongs in her role. If the manager learns to manage conflict with competence, he will start to see himself as a leader. If the founder's daughter learns the business, maintains or improves the company culture, and demonstrates her commitment to the organization, she will be seen as the heir apparent. None of that will happen automatically, however. It will take effort and commitment and time.

Go back and look through this chapter. Which fears resonate most with you? Can you identify one or two that really seem to hold you back? Which examples or stories could have been taken from your own life?

In Chapter 8, you are going to be asked to think about the fears that keep you from being the person you want to be, so you might as well start identifying them now. Before that, however, we will focus on how to adjust your mindset in order to deal with fear. Sometimes your attitude can make all of the difference in the world.

Takeaways:

- Even though we have gone through numerous models of fears, including Albrecht's feararchy, these are not necessarily what plague us in everyday life. The more realistic and tangible fears we are facing typically have to do with social constructs.
- Perhaps the most powerful fear we hold and live by is the fear of failure and rejection. This is powerful because it can create an effect where we wish to avoid failure and rejection; thus, we do nothing, because that gives us a 100% chance of avoiding that negative feeling. This is known as learned helplessness. The only solution here is to reframe how you view

failure and rejection—it doesn't cause the end of the world, and it can be your best teacher.

- The second truly commonplace fear is the fear of judgment. This is another social fear. We care far too much what people think about us and let it dictate our decisions. We are skewed to believe that we are perpetually in the spotlight, which is patently untrue. We let this all affect our self-worth, which means we define ourselves by the perception of others, not ourselves. Often, a cost-benefit analysis will reveal that the fear of judgment is negligible, while the life you are missing out on is unfortunately massive.

- The third fear we face is the fear of change and the unknown. Like fear itself, change is neutral, but we always think about the worst-case scenario and fear that we are making a grave mistake. Attempt to switch your focus from all the possible obstacles to everything that is currently going right. If all else fails, find support and comfort in the factors of your life that won't ever change.

- The final fear we face is the fear of success, which sounds paradoxical. The truth is, many of us don't like the ancillary effects that success brings, such as increased attention and expectations. People don't want to be put under scrutiny and thus are prone to self-sabotage.

Chapter 4. Shift Your Mindset

By this point, it should be clear that fear is a natural human reaction; fear itself is not bad. The problem with fear is how people deal with it. When fear affects relationships, goals, moving forward, and well-being, it cannot be ignored.

Thirty years ago, Stanford brain researcher Carol Dweck coined the phrases *fixed mindset* and *growth mindset*. She used these terms to help define how people respond to failure— whether they are devastated or whether they can bounce back. People who have a growth mindset have a belief that they can improve, grow, and change, while people with a fixed mindset believe everyone has predetermined limitations. You can guess which one is more effective at tackling fear.

Changing your mindset, your core beliefs, about how you deal with fear can make a huge impact on your ability to manage your fears. And while it is not as easy as clapping your hands and chanting "I do believe in fairies, I do believe in fairies," the results can be just as remarkable. When your attitude says, "I can overcome this fear," then the likelihood of you actually doing it is far greater than if you repeatedly tell yourself that you are doomed to live with your fears forever.

The Victim Mentality

A common characteristic of people who live with fear is a concept known as *victim mentality*.

The victim mentality causes people to perceive that they have no power over their own actions or circumstances. This is not a new story; it goes all the way back to the biblical fall of man. Adam blamed Eve for giving him the forbidden fruit; Eve blamed the serpent for persuading her to take it. It is the age-old story of *the devil made me do it*— people claiming to be powerless instead of taking responsibility. Taking on the role of the victim is actually a response to fear. People who live thinking the universe is against them perceive the universe to be a very scary and horrible thing.

People who struggle with the victim mentality are convinced life is not only beyond their control, but that it is also deliberately out to hurt them. This belief results in constant blame, finger-pointing, and pity parties that are fueled by pessimism, anger, and fear. Disempowering self-talk takes control and people blame others, bemoan circumstances, and engage in self-pity. Nearly everyone knows someone who is constantly saying, "If only this would happen, things would be better" or "Why her and not me?" or "If I were in charge, we would do it this way."

David Emerald, in his book *Power of TED,* calls this victim mentality the "dreaded drama triangle" after a concept developed in the 1960s by Dr. Steven Karpman. People stuck in the victim mentality play any, or all, of the three roles: victims, persecutors, or rescuers.

As **victims,** people focus on everything negative in their lives. They blame everything bad that happens to them on someone or something else. They do not take responsibility for their own actions, and they rarely see any connection between their actions and the consequences. They feel wronged by those who criticize or judge them.

As **persecutors,** people judge and criticize others, typically from a place of anger and spite. They are the ones making statements like "This is all your fault" or "Why didn't you make a plan for this." Interestingly, sometimes, perhaps even often, the victim and the persecutor are same person.

Finally, people turn to **rescuers**, which could be another person, a vice, or some other distraction, for relief. Perhaps you are more familiar with the word *enabler*. The rescuer is the one who gives the person permission to fail. Often, they are motived by their own desire to swoop in and save the day. The rescuer makes the victim dependent.

For example, Gail, our constant victim, is single and struggles with feeling lonely. She often refers to the "one who got away" because her father disapproved of their relationship. She blames her father for the fact she is alone. She has a friend, Anne, who has experienced some success with online dating, but instead of trying it herself, Gail, who is now serving as her own persecutor, mocks Anne and dismisses online dating as shallow. She justifies her daily habit of having a large dessert, the vice that is the rescuer in this case, before bed as a way of comforting herself. Gail is caught in the drama triangle. Because she is in this trap, she never deals with the real problem, the fear of being alone.

Emerald's antidote to this drama triangle is called "the empowerment dynamic." Instead of victims, persecutors, and rescuers, the characters in this situation are creators, challengers, and coaches.

Where victims focus on problems, **creators** focus on what they want. They become empowered to create outcomes for their own lives. They have the same problems, challenges, and life events as victims; they just view them through a different lens. Instead of persecutors, **challengers** help creators learn and grow throughout their journey of self-exploration.

Finally, instead of rescuers, creators have **coaches** who are supportive as the creator moves toward the desired outcome. They don't allow negativity to fester and can shine the light on the correct or better path. This approach allows people to face their fears, instead of passively letting bad things to happen, by allowing other people help along the way.

Consider a different approach Gail could take. Even though she is single and often feels lonely, Gail has decided to let go of her past relationship mistakes and focus on building new relationships. Her friend, Anne, offers to help her meet some people through various organizations. After some exploration, Gail decides she wants to volunteer at a local elementary school. While working at the school, she meets Frank, the school principal, who encourages her to consider a more active role within the school.

He connects Gail with a group of volunteers who plan literacy events with the school librarian. Gail enjoys the fulfillment of volunteering with the children and builds some good relationships with the other volunteers. A small group of them regularly meet for coffee even when they are not planning an event. In this scenario Gail is the creator, Anne is the challenger, and Frank and the other volunteers are the coaches.

While there is no guarantee, Gail's actions in the second scenario have several very positive results. First, Gail becomes the one in control. By taking a few concrete actions, she is not simply allowing the universe to feed her sense of loneliness. Second, she is not passing judgments on her friend. By allowing Anne to challenge her to do something new that may or may not be within her comfort zone, Gail demonstrates respect for her friend. Finally, by stepping out, Gail is meeting new people who are helping her discover new talents and interests while providing new relationships to ease her initial issue of feeling lonely.

A change in mindset truly can result in a change in circumstance, and often people can unwittingly find themselves playing the victim. By focusing on your best qualities and believing you can have the things you want, you can change your mindset and become more comfortable tackling your fears.

Inferiority Complex

Changing your mindset can also change your attitude toward your fears. As people become more comfortable trying to overcome their fears, their confidence grows. Confidence, however, can be difficult to achieve for those who struggle with feeling inferior.

The famous psychologist Alfred Adler once said that feeling inferior is often a healthy motivator. His argument was that if individuals receive criticism or see another person doing something better than them, then they are driven to eliminate their own weaknesses. In other words, feeling inferior causes people to learn from superior people around them, and it motivates them to want to improve themselves. Thus, they will put in the necessary work to develop themselves and become confident.

Adler also recognized, however, that some people take feelings of inferiority too far—indeed, to the point it is no longer healthy, useful, or inspiring. Adler called this an *inferiority complex*. Instead of motivating, an inferiority complex paralyzes. It can result in extreme shyness, social anxiety, feelings of worthlessness, and the desire to avoid failure by not trying.

This should sound familiar. The fear of failure is one of the top things people fear. Often, that fear of failure is directly linked to an inferiority complex—that feeling of never being as good as others—even though the person believes he or she should be as good as others. A person with an inferiority complex might not think she is smart enough to show her boss she deserves a promotion. Instead of increasing her own knowledge or building her skill set, she gets trapped by her fear of failure and remains stagnant.

People who feel inferior tend to think in terms of "all or nothing." When they are not as good as others, they struggle to understand why that is. *Utopianism* is a term used to identify "if only" thinking. People come to believe if only this would happen, they would be better.

"If only I would 20 pounds, I would be more attractive. If only I made more money, I would be less stressed. If only I had a child, I would feel more fulfilled." Unfortunately, life's "if onlys" rarely do little more than provide temporary relief to ongoing issues. For the most part, people who are trapped into believing these "if only" statements already know what they should do, but because of their fear, they avoid it.

If you really believe you would be more attractive if you weighed 20 fewer pounds, then why don't you lose weight? There are plenty of fears that keep people from shedding pounds: fear of failure, fear of missing out on some comfort from food, fear of injury while exercising, fear of embarrassment while exercising, fear of losing weight and then being asked on a date, fear of only being liked because of your figure. The list of fears is endless, all premised on the fact that you just don't believe you're worthy or capable.

To overcome an inferiority complex, it is necessary to have a shift in thinking about what prevents you from feeling confident. By systematically combating distorted thinking patterns about personal flaws, people can start to fix the problem. It is essential to realize no flaw is as bad as you think; having weaknesses is a part of the human experience. Realizing that everyone has some flaws, and most people have major flaws, allows a person to recognize this is a phenomenon we all face. Finally, realizing that having certain flaws does not mean you do not have talents or desirable qualities.

When a person who has a fear of failure also struggles with an inferiority complex, the key to overcoming the fear is to build confidence up so that failure does not seem frightening. Remember, failure is part of life; it can be a learning experience. Failing prepares us for success. However, a person who constantly tells herself "I am not good enough, and therefore I will fail" is like a buffering YouTube video—stuck.

There are many ways people identify themselves as inferior. Some people focus on their perceived defects: "I'm not good enough. I'm a bad person. I'm a failure." Others focus on perception of being unlovable: "Nobody wants me. I'm always left out." Still another group considers themselves with no power or control: "I am trapped. I cannot measure up to others. There is no way out." Notice how similar these thoughts of inferiority are to the fears mentioned in Chapter 3. The things we fear the most are things about which we are most vulnerable. If you continually feel inferior, this colors everything in life to be an opportunity for failure because you just don't think success is in the cards for you.

Amor Fati

In order to move past some common fears about the situations life can bring, German philosopher Friedrich Nietzsche provides some insight on how to be satisfied with what life dishes out.

> *"My formula for what is great in mankind is* amor fati: *not to wish for anything other than that which is; whether behind, ahead, or for all eternity. Not just to put up with the inevitable—much less to hide it from oneself, for all idealism is lying to oneself in the face of the necessary— but to love it."*

Amor fati, which literally means the love of fate, simply means to accept and love everything that happens. In other words, Nietzsche offers the key to a happy life: do not wish for reality to be any different; rather, accept and love whatever happens.

Some things are going to happen that will a create fear response. There is no way around it. Nietzsche's advice is to simply accept the situation as it is—no wishing it away or agonizing over it. When you agonize over something, you are causing yourself to suffer twice—with the ruminating and the actual event, if it even occurs.

Consider the ancient metaphor of being leashed to a cart: the *wise* man is like a dog leashed to a moving cart, running joyfully alongside and smoothly keeping pace with it; the *foolish* man is like a dog that struggles against the leash but finds himself dragged beside the cart anyway. Both dogs are in the same situation, but which one has the better journey and feels less resistance and more happiness? Obviously, it is the one who does not fight what he cannot beat.

We have the option of going along and enjoying the ride, or we have the option of fighting and complaining all the way. Since nobody wants to be dragged along, the best thing we can do is make the most of the journey and plan for the journey itself rather than fuss about how bad it might be. Nietzsche would advise us to embrace fear, even when it is paralyzing—because what else is there to do from a fatalistic standpoint?

Complaining will not help, and pulling away will not help, but moving forward and facing what comes allows us to experience all sorts of terrain: joy, love, excitement, boredom, sadness, and, yes, even fear. The key is to keep going forward, along for the ride, no matter what we face.

Does this sound like you are simply caving to fear? Just because people try to love what happens does not mean they condone or approve of it. It simply means they understand they cannot change it, so the best option is to accept it and try to make the best of it. Then people can identify the best action to take in the situation—something wholly missing if you choose to focus on how bad it will be. By embracing fate, we embrace our failures, our success, our powerlessness—all of those things we find terrifying and immobilizing.

The idea is simple: take every moment as it is; take reality as it is; do not resist or it will have power over you; if you take it as it comes, it will have no power over you. It is a simple idea but difficult to put into practice. One way to put this philosophy into action is by recognizing that things come and go.

Vernon Howard offers the following: "We can see that our pain lies between what we think should happen and what actually happens. Then, if we remove the secret demand for this or that to happen, the pain-gap vanishes."

The concept of *amor fati*, accepting and loving whatever fate brings to life, allows people to develop a life philosophy that almost laughs in the face of fear. Instead of being afraid of the unknown, embrace it. Instead of fearing failure, accept it. Instead of worrying about the judgment of others, let it roll off without giving it any consideration at all.

The question still exists, however: how does a person love fate when fate sometimes brings negative things? For example, when fate brings a job loss, how can that be something to love? Or when fate results in a relationship ending, how can that be something to love?

Loving fate does not mean celebrating when something horrible happens but shifting your mindset to look past it and adapt. Whether you are learning to be more independent, learning to speak up for yourself, or learning to take control of something that felt out of control, you will be standing up to your old adversary, fear.

Consider the loss of a job. It is one of those situations that people fear will happen and then are they are filled with fear when it does happen. It makes people feel inferior to others. Additionally, there are serious and fear-inducing consequences of a job loss. On all fronts, it is a horrible situation.

By embracing *amor fati*, you would accept the loss and move on to whatever fate brings. Perhaps it becomes a chance to explore a new job focus; perhaps it is a catalyst for starting that small business that up until now was only a daydream; perhaps it is the motivation to return for additional training or education.

In any case, there is no way to move backward or even stay stagnant, so your only choice is to embrace the present and move forward.

Sound scary? It probably will be. Your fears are what will prevent you from living this way, if you let them. Instead of allowing fear to dictate your attitude toward fate, fearlessly take fate as it comes.

Taking Calculated Risks

Fear is unavoidable, but humans can't help but ruminate and blow it out of proportion. Therefore, it is important to assess fear and risk in an accurate manner. By doing this we can learn to base fears on reality rather than on emotions—emotions are the downfall here.

The human mind does not like unknowns. Unknowns throw a wrench into the system. When your mind comes to an unknown, it makes up an answer. Where experience lacks, the brain glosses right over and fills in the blank with its own answer to the question, *what happens next*? Usually, what's filled in is something unrealistically tragic because the part of the brain that creates the answer is the amygdala, the part of the brain that processes fear.

Therefore, without even realizing it, people take a worthwhile endeavor and label it too risky without even realizing that the process through which that determination was made was inherently flawed. Probability and reality be damned.

Thanks to the amygdala, the equation contained the wrong numbers and it was rigged to fail before it got started. Suddenly something that we have no experience with is frightening. Instead of making an honest, well-considered appraisal of the situation, we have allowed our auto pilot to give us bad information, and it almost always stimulates the fear response in us.

There is a better way than to let your amygdala run the show. No question, life is filled with risks. But it's not nearly as scary as you would believe.

A calculated risk is an act that is pursued after a careful consideration of the risks. Generally speaking, a calculated risk is taken after the decision has been made that the potential rewards of an action outweigh the risk. Several factors that influence a person about whether or not to take certain calculated risks include their own level of risk tolerance and the availability of less-risky alternatives. The task is to put your fears into an accurate perspective.

Asking what the risks are and then seeking an honest answer is necessary. People cannot allow their emotions to prevent them from carefully considering all the risks and seeing them accurately. Buying a fixer-upper hotel on the beach sounds exciting. The temptation of owning a place where families come for fun would make a wonderful life. It could also be a landmine. Reel in the excitement, and take some time to research.

Also, just because something sounds great, though, does not mean it is too good to be true. While investing your life's savings without doing any research is probably too risky, it is also important to avoid fixating on the negative possibilities and catastrophizing every scenario, as this will make a person more risk-averse. There does have to be balance between gathering good information and remaining convinced that everything holds too much risk.

Consider this example. You could take a trip and have eight-hour delays at the airport, lost luggage, a dirty hotel room, and a case of Montezuma's revenge after eating at the buffet. If you are afraid that taking time off from your job might jeopardize that promotion you're trying to snag, then you could scare yourself out of a much-needed vacation.

When considering risks, think about the odds of the risk becoming true. Be truthful about this. Use real data by doing research and talking to others. This is where many people are guilty of inflating the probability of negative outcomes and making things that are not actually risky seem dangerous. When considering the rewards, be sensible. Use real evidence and not simply assumptions. Find out how many others have done something similar and how they have fared. By discovering the true probability, the true worst-case scenario, and the true possible rewards, people can learn to take calculated risks.

Going back to the example of a job loss, during the time when a person is making a decision about what to do next, there will be plenty of opportunities to evaluate risks and rewards. Consider Kate, who lost her job as an administrative assistant when her company was trimming the fat. Kate had multiple options, including looking for another job, returning to school to finish her degree in accounting, or trying something totally new.

During her decision-making process, one of the ideas Kate came up with was starting her own business as a virtual personal assistant. It was easy to come up with a list of risks that could have prevented her from trying. She also considered the rewards, which for her were really positive: the ability to control her own workload, the chance to make more money, and the flexibility to be able to work from almost anywhere.

Even though the rewards made it tempting to jump in with both feet, she knew that was too risky. She did a lot of research about what could go right and what could go wrong during the process of getting her business up and running.

After careful consideration of all of her research, she decided the potential benefits of working for herself outweighed the possible risks; in other words, the calculated risk was low enough that she could move forward. Because she had done good research, she understood the true probability of her success, and thanks to her ever-active amygdala, she had imagined multiple worst-case scenario options. Luckily, she could see that those catastrophes were unlikely to happen. She put her fears in their place by doing the work she needed to understand exactly what she was getting into.

The example of Kate makes taking a calculated risk seem easy. For most people, even with all of the facts, deciding to take a risk is, well, risky. What is important to remember, though, is that fear keeps people from taking risks, even ones that hold the potential for great benefits. You can live with fear ruling your life, or you can rule your life yourself. You have to be smart and thoughtful, but you don't have to be afraid of taking a calculated risk, especially if things are in your favor.

Go back to the first paragraph of this chapter and reread the difference between a fixed mindset and a growth mindset. Realize that they are instrumental to how you view the world and how fear affects you. In the next chapter, we will focus on how your inner monologue affects your mindset and what you can do to change it.

Takeaways

- The mindset we have regarding fear can color our entire world. The perception of mindset as an important element of success was first proposed by Carol Dweck, who found differences between growth and fixed mindsets.
- As far as how it relates to fear, a mindset to avoid is the victim mentality. This is where you feel that you have no control about what's happening to you, and you necessarily view everything as a plot designed to bring you down. Obviously, this makes fear even worse because it feels inevitable and unstoppable.
- Another mindset to adjust is the inferiority complex, which is when you simply feel that you are not good enough or worthy of good things happening. This contributes to fear because it creates fear out of thin air, even when you should feel confident.
- A mindset to start embodying is *amor fati*, which translates to love of fate. When you can abide by this, you can embrace and love when something fearful or negative

happens to you, recognizing that it is neutral and you can turn it into something positive—at the least, something neutral. You are not giving up or accepting mediocrity; you are simply moving past the present and thinking about how to proceed after the fact.

- A final mindset to learn is that of taking calculated risks. This is difficult in the face of fear because we can't help but think emotionally and irrationally. Thus, we ignore statistics and probabilities and make poor decisions. Attempt to remain even-keeled and objectively evaluate risk so the presence of fear isn't making you reactionary.

Chapter 5. Choose Your Inner Monologue

The inner monologue is the voice inside your head that tells you how to feel about the world. The way people talk to themselves can either create more fear and doubt or it can give them the courage to face whatever may come. Your inner monologue is what you tell yourself; it is constantly running and not always in our control. It can be positive or negative; it has the power to give or destroy a person's confidence.

Do you start your morning with the words "I'm ready to face the day" or "I wish it wasn't morning"?

When you are asked to do something extra at work is your first thought "That's not my job" or "I'm glad she trusts me with this"? Your inner monologue dictates your perception about life and how you will feel in various situations. Of course, it can also affect how you deal with the aspects of your life that conjure fear.

When you need to make a difficult phone call, what do you tell yourself? "I'm sure this will go terribly." "I know she will be angry." "I hope I don't start to cry." If you do, you are only reinforcing your own fears. In this chapter, we will explore how changing your inner monologue, your self-talk, into a tool that helps you beat your fears.

We've talked about how fear's purpose is to provide information about the scenario at hand. Remember, fear is our body's way of protecting us from things that are dangerous. It is not meant to keep people from having fun or enjoying life; sadly, however, when people do not learn to manage their fear, it can do just that. When you overperceive the presence of fear, your inner monologue immediately shifts into protection mode and turns a field of flowers into a field of hidden landmines and imminent harm.

Consider the example of being invited to meet someone for a coffee date. However, because you have not dated anyone since your last serious relationship ended in spectacular fashion, you are a bit skittish about going. Simply being in a romantic context sets your alarm bells off. Whereas your inner monologue might be more forgiving if you hadn't had that experience— "This is such a great opportunity to meet someone"—because you perceive fear, the voice inside your head gives you a very different take: "This might not be such a good idea. Remember what happened last time? You can't deal with that again so soon."

Your inner monologue can completely change your perspective on a potential event. Most of the time, it will probably influence whether you take action or not. This seems like being sentenced to prison by something that you can't control, but the inner monologue can be a conscious choice. Reframing that inner monologue can give you just the boost of confidence you need to overcome a fear-inducing situation.

Fearful or Excited?

As stated above, one of the greatest reasons for utilizing your inner monologue as a tool for overcoming fear is the fact that we get to choose the words we say to ourselves.

The first step of changing your inner monologue is to realize that fear is often accompanied by other emotions—most commonly excitement. Think of riding a roller coaster or seeing a horror movie. Both of those activities can be seriously frightening, but they are also exhilarating. A life without fear and the thrill of overcoming fear would be bland and insipid. Feeling afraid when trying something new or challenging is natural. It is also natural to experience joy and excitement while stretching yourself and facing those fears.

And that's what we are going to take advantage of in changing our inner monologue. Instead of seeing things through the lens of fear, see things through the lens of excitement, thrill, and achievement. You can acknowledge fear, but choose to focus on how a situation might challenge you and make you grow.

"I can't ride a roller coaster because I might faint" sounds like someone who is terrified, while "I want to ride the roller coaster **because** it makes me feel like I might faint" sounds like someone who is eager. The sentence has changed just slightly, but the meaning is completely different. You can choose to say something that reinforces your fear response and keeps you stuck where you are, or you can choose to encourage yourself and experience the joy and excitement of embracing a new challenge.

Bungee jumping is one of those extreme sports that most people consider too far out there, yet everyday people around the world line up to do it. In Macau, people pay over $500 USD to leap 764 feet off the Macau

Tower, the world's highest bungee jump. How might you approach this through excitement and not fear?

If the inner chatter includes things like "I can't do this. I won't survive. I am not strong enough," then they will turn around, unbuckle the harness, and take the elevator. Yet those who hear their inner voice saying words like "I'm going to do this. I'm going to fall and bounce and scream and laugh all the way down, but I'm doing this because it is insane" allow themselves to drop toward the ground and take in the rush.

This is certainly not a suggestion that everyone needs to run out and try leaping off buildings, but imagine the power that staring a fear in the face gives someone. "If I am brave enough to jump off a building, surely I can speak with my boss about a promotion." Doing something terrifying and surviving it makes people feel empowered.

Your inner monologue can give you the power to jump, and it can give you words to tell yourself later whenever you feel scared in the future. The only way this will work, however, is if you embrace an inner monologue that says, "Go for it." When you tell yourself that, you choose excitement over fear.

Similarly, achieving something difficult teaches people they have the fortitude it takes to see things through to the end. Committing to a physical challenge like running a race or competing in a triathlon is scary because it forces us to put our pride on the line. However, after training and completing a challenge like that, people not only overcome their fears, but they also see themselves in a new way.

Instead of falling back on the old inner monologue of "I am not committed to completing this degree because I am lazy and don't want to work," change it to "If I am strong enough to run a 10K, I can finish my dissertation." The inner monologue can allow you to reframe your perceptions about yourself and about the tasks in front of you.

Rather than being fearful about laziness, become excited about perseverance. It's a choice that is difficult at first to make and may even feel silly and pointless. But it's not like your fear system knows the difference.

Permission to Fear

Another part of the inner monologue to change is how feeling fear itself is viewed. Being fearful is perfectly normal. In fact, in many situations, it would be unusual, even abnormal, for a person to have no fears.

Some people equate feeling fear with being cowardly. When they are in a situation that feels frightening, their inner monologue continues to focus on the negative. Telling themselves things like "If I were a stronger person, this would not frighten me" or "Normal people are not afraid of every little challenge that comes along" will only reinforce the idea that fear is not normal. Of course, that just creates a cycle where you feel bad, you tell yourself you should feel bad for feeling bad, and then you feel worse. Rinse and repeat.

There is no reason to resist negative emotions by denying and repressing them. There is no reason to feel guilty or ashamed for experiencing certain emotions. See emotions for what they are and deal with them appropriately.

To do that, make sure you are speaking to yourself in the appropriate way. Your inner monologue can say, "This is scary." That's natural and acceptable. But it turns into a problem when you begin to add onto that statement, such as, "Because this is scary, I cannot handle it." You do not need to deny the existence of your fear, but you can use your inner monologue to convince yourself that you have the courage to deal with it. When you give yourself permission to feel fear and understand that it's a natural part of the process, it becomes much more manageable and acceptable.

One area where a lot of people struggle with confidence is in public speaking. It is easy to look at someone who seems to fit into the spotlight naturally and think that speaking in public has never been an issue for her. That does not mean they don't still sometimes feel anxious or afraid when speaking up. It just means they have learned, thanks to their budding confidence, how to control those very normal feelings. They have learned that it is a part of the process, and the presence of fear doesn't actually mean anything negative.

Fear is neutral, remember? Therefore, fear is just a part of public speaking, like climbing the stairs to the stage and being used to staring into a bright spotlight. Everyone feels fear, and you should always factor it in your expectations.

Reappraisal

While giving yourself permission to feel fear can improve your ability to handle it, other approaches that are less direct can also help.

Sometimes the best thing a person can do is simply change the way she looks at fear. Perhaps giving a slightly different interpretation to fear—for example, calling it something other than fear—can make all the difference. For instance, instead of repeating to yourself that you are afraid, repeat to yourself you are extremely cautious. While at first this could sound like excuse-making, again, your brain doesn't know the difference and will listen to what it's told. If it is told that there is no fear and only caution, guess what you will feel?

The trick is to learn when cautiousness is a real and genuine protection and when it is your go-to excuse for avoidance. Consider this study that offers a way to reframe your thinking.

Reappraisal was coined by Oschner and Gross in 2008. The classic definition for reappraisal is to look at something in a new or different manner. It is commonly used in the mortgage industry when someone wants to refinance their house. They often reappraise, or appraise it again, based on the current market to see if there have been changes since the last appraisal (or judgment or assessment) was made.

In applying reappraisal to psychology, Ochsner's study showed participants a photo of people crying outside a church. The participants first reported feelings of sadness. Then participants were asked to imagine the scene was at a wedding and the photos were of people crying tears of joy. Using an MRI, it was possible to see the brains of the participants change at the moment they reappraised the situation.

Ochsner explains, "Our emotional responses ultimately flow out of our appraisals of the world, and if we shift those appraisals, we shift our emotional responses." That means we can reappraise or even relabel a situation to manipulate how we feel about it. Whatever we tell ourselves about a situation truly lets us feel differently about it. If we simply weave a story where fear is not present, we will feel substantially less fear.

Reappraisal is a tool that can allow people to diminish or eliminate certain fears. For some people, the sentence "We need to talk" strikes fear. They immediately imagine something is wrong or they are going to need to justify something. Instead of thinking, "Something must be wrong," reframing the thought to "He must want my advice" or "He needs me to clarify something" can change the outlook on the upcoming conversation. When something initially strikes fear, a reappraisal may be what's needed to put the situation into perspective and remove the presence of fear.

Another example of effective use of reappraisal is when faced with a medical scare. Some people automatically think the words "further tests" can only mean "further tests to **confirm** something horrible." A reappraisal of the thoughts to "further tests to **rule out** something horrible" will not have any bearing on the actual outcome of the tests, but it can help calm fears and improve a person's outlook.

Reappraisal allows you to rid yourself of worst-case scenarios. It allows you to see other possibilities that might not be so bad. That can help reduce fear or increase courage in facing the fear. When reappraisal becomes a habit, you can start to see the silver lining among the storm clouds. In order for that to happen, you have to make a choice to direct your inner monologue.

Prudent vs. Fearful

In the last section, there was brief mention of when acting on fear is cautious rather than fearful. Let's take another look at that. We've established that fear has a purpose: to keep us safe and warn us of danger. Being *prudent* means we heed that warning and take action to avoid the potential danger.

A person's inner monologue is essential in helping decide what actions are prudent, but remember, your inner monologue is something you choose to tell yourself. When something just doesn't feel right and that nagging won't go away, it is prudent to examine why. You are acting responsibly and analyzing what your caveman instincts are trying to tell you.

It's possible you are simply avoiding action or making a decision because of a fear, but it's also possible you are getting a legitimate warning. It can be difficult to tell the difference sometimes. Are you facing an irrational fear or being prudent? Shift your inner monologue and use your analytical skills to decide the answer to that question. Perhaps someone showed up on your doorstep selling investment life-insurance policies. Even if you are seriously interested in the product, good judgment (that is prudence) would guide your inner monologue to "I need to do some research. I want to gather some data. If it sounds too good to be true, it might be."

A person's inner monologue is essential in removing irrational and unreasonable fears. For example, you might be afraid to make an important phone call because your inner monologue says that if it does not go well, you will be seen as a failure. One phone call and you are a failure at your work or your relationship? Surely not. Choose to change your inner monologue and overcome that fear. In this example, your inner monologue is using prudence as an excuse to avoid something difficult. In other words, being prudent is actually an excuse to avoid an irrational fear.

While irrational fears can hold people back and keep them from finding success, other fears could be realistic, and heeding them is simply good judgment. For example, a person who is afraid of driving after having a couple of drinks, even though she does not feel drunk, is actually showing responsibility. A person who chooses not to alter the books because he is afraid of being arrested is demonstrating a strong code of ethics. Prudence is always a good thing.

Deciding what is maintaining an irrational fear and what is being prudent can be tricky. The problem, though, is most often in the reverse. People claim something is prudence when in reality it is an irrational fear.

For example, refusing to go on a date because you do not want to risk heartbreak is irrational. First, if one date leads to heartbreak, then the expectations for the date were completely out of line. Second, a date has the potential to lead to a relationship or to nowhere, plus a lot of nuances in between. There is no reason to assume it will automatically lead to heartbreak. Going on one date with someone is rarely a risk, especially when trying to avoid heartbreak.

Learning to use that inner monologue to remind yourself of what is irrational and what is prudent is an important part of overcoming irrational fears, which often stand in the way of what people really want.

Sometimes, it can be just as easy as asking some questions: "What am I really afraid of? Am I trying to avoid something that really is a possible outcome or am I trying to avoid something that is unlikely to be an outcome?" Learning to answer those questions honestly about fears can help a person discover where to take risks and move forward. Remember, labeling yourself as prudent doesn't make it so. Real prudence is the result of making decisions carefully without making excuses and of reframing yourself in that mold as opposed to being fearful of everything that comes your way. You are Sherlock Holmes, not someone cowering under the blanket.

Your inner monologue has to line up with what you want out of life. If it does not, you will be doomed to stay right where you are and be held back by the voice inside your head.

Fear is a mindset that frequently occurs because of how we talk to ourselves. By allowing yourself to get excited about new challenges, things that were frightening become invigorating. By remembering that fear is natural, we don't spiral out of control. Using a tool like reappraisal can help you evaluate your fears and determine whether your response is one of fear or one of prudence. There is never an expectation of instantly becoming mentally tough, but we tend to feel what people tell us. Use this to your advantage.

Takeaways:

- Your inner monologue is the little voice inside your head that tells you to beware, be careful, and overall fear what comes your way. But, it can be changed. Your inner monologue doesn't have to take that angle—we should strive to improve it so it can empower us, not disempower us.

- The first way to change our inner monologues is to choose for the voice to dwell on excitement versus fear. Excitement and fear are often two sides of the same coin, but one of them promotes a positive attitude, while the other makes you cower and want to retreat.

- The second way to change our inner monologues is to give yourself permission to feel fear. The presence of fear is not a failure, nor it is uncommon. It is a natural part of any process. Therefore, if fear is present, take it as a sign that you are on the right path instead of the feeling that something is deeply wrong with you.

- The third way to change our inner monologues is to practice reappraisal, which is the act of framing a fearful act in a silver lining type of way. Studies have shown that simply relabeling something drastically changes how we feel about it, and we can do the same thing for fear.

- The fourth way to change our inner monologues is to choose prudence over fear. Instead of being fearful, you are being smart, cautious, and prudent. Again, when you harp on emotions other than fear, fear tends to fade. Just make sure this doesn't become a convenient excuse for yourself.

Chapter 6. The Case for Action

Talking about fears and thinking about fears can be helpful, but at some level, that may not be enough to get a person over the hump. Sometimes the thing that is needed is simple action, even if infinitesimal at first. After all, Rome wasn't built in a day, and your fears cannot be extracted or managed in a day.

Action can build confidence because it allows people to understand that fears exist mostly because of ignorance and a lack of exposure. No matter how scary it is, that little tiny leap of faith is required to spark confidence and the knowledge that what you fear won't kill you.

The ancient philosopher Aristotle, who focused many of his teachings on courage, said that people develop courage by performing courageous acts. Practicing courage, according to Aristotle, can make all the difference in life.

The case for action in beating fear is quite strong. Let's be clear that we aren't necessarily talking about conquering and defeating a fear—that is a much longer process that may never end. Instead, this chapter focuses on taking *fearless action,* which allows you to bypass the puzzle of how to approach a fear by simply diving in. Living fearlessly requires a split second, a leap of faith. Personally, I'd opt for that path to the life I want instead of endlessly planning and rationalizing everything first.

It turns out, contrary to what others would have you believe, we can't simply *logic* fear out of existence-at least not at a speed that you'd be happy with. Fear is not a logical emotion, and you can't reason with it. It doesn't listen to your arguments and will steamroll you unless you have a competing emotion to quell it. It's like the dog that just won't listen to your commands despite being trained for years. Therefore, *action and doing* and the subsequent small victories that ensue are necessary for beating fear.

Become Fearless

Becoming fearless is not easy.

As most suggestions are, some will be more appealing than others; in fact, some of them can become excuses to procrastinate. For example, one such reason is research and planning. Doing thorough and thoughtful research is essential to the good decision-making process. However, research and planning can sometimes act as a buffer between you and the discomfort of action.

At the beginning of this journey, you are never going to feel that you are fully ready to take the first foray out of your comfort zone, but that's just the thing. You can't wait until you feel like you have built up all of your confidence and feel that things will go 100% your way, because that moment will never come. You'll be stuck waiting forever.

If you want to skydive, then at some point you just have to jump. There's no amount of rumination or preparation that will truly make you feel confident in jumping out of a flying piece of metal with only a parachute strapped to your back. You have no idea how it feels, so there's just no way you can accurately prepare. It's the successful completion of small, medium, and large actions that build your confidence. Therefore, beating fear works in an opposite order as what feels safe for us.

How many times have you withheld doing something you wanted because you wanted to wait until the day you felt fully confident to do it? The problem with this tendency toward feeling safe is your confidence will never increase unless you do the thing that you are avoiding. Ironically, that is exactly what will build it. And when you do it time after time, that's when fear really starts to subside. Make mistakes of action, not inaction, and force yourself to take action precisely when you feel scared and uncomfortable, because that is the only approach that will truly work.

A note: it's important to focus on the action itself, not whether there was a positive outcome. You can control taking a step out of your comfort zone, but you can't necessarily control what the outcome might be—at first.

Fearlessness is the ability to do something despite the fact that you are terrified of it. Fearlessness ignores all negative consequences, while confidence is the understanding that negative consequences will be acceptable and unlikely. People would be more successful if they were to aim for fearlessness rather than outright confidence, because fearlessness gets more done.

Fearlessness allows you to jump off a building or approach someone attractive because you only need to suspend fear for 10 seconds. Confidence doesn't necessarily allow you to do this. And most importantly, fearlessness allows you to take action sooner rather than later.

Defeating fear begins outside of your comfort zone. The reason you are reading this book is your comfort zone is too small, so you feel anxious more than you'd like. You have to continually take steps outside of your comfort zone to keep expanding it, or you'll be right where you started. As the saying goes, if you keep doing what you've been doing, you'll keep getting the results you've been getting. Nothing will change, and nothing will improve.

Full confidence in every situation is impossible to achieve. You could spend an entire lifetime and never achieve it. Fearlessness requires just a moment of faith in yourself.

As fear is removed, confidence does tend to emerge. People who have a strong sense of confidence believe results will be positive, while people who live with fear worry about potential negative results. Once the fear of a negative result is gone, it is much easier to believe that a positive result will come. The problem is, confidence will not be there in every situation, so sometimes, the best option is to take the plunge.

Does this mean every time a person is faced with a scary situation she should immediately take a leap and go for it? Actually, trying to live fearlessly all of the time is not much healthier than living paralyzed by fear. No surprise, balance is key. Thinking things through can be important; it is important to note, though, that not everything needs to be thought through to multiple conclusions.

The 40–70 Rule

Many of us are reluctant to take action toward fear unless we have all the pertinent information we need about it. But can you actually have *too* much information to start something new?

Former U.S. Secretary of State Colin Powell has a rule of thumb about making decisions and coming to a point of action. He says that any time you face a hard choice, you should have *no less* than 40% and *no more* than 70% of the information you need to make that decision. In that range, you have enough information to make an informed choice but not so much intelligence that you lose your resolve and simply stay abreast of the situation.

If you have less than 40% of the information you need, you're essentially shooting from the hip. You don't know quite enough to move forward and will probably make a lot of mistakes. Conversely, if you chase down more data until you get more than 70% of what you need (and it's unlikely that you'll truly need anything above this level), you could get overwhelmed and uncertain. The opportunity may have passed you by, and someone else may have beaten you by starting already.

But in that sweet spot between 40% and 70%, you have enough to go on and let your intuition guide your decisions. In the context of Colin Powell, this is where effective leaders are made: the ones who have instincts that point in the right direction are who will lead their organizations to success.

For our purposes of breaking out of the comfort zone, we can replace the word "information" with other motivators: 40–70% of experience, 40–70% reading or learning, 40–70% confidence, or 40–70% of planning. While we're completing the task, we'll also be doing analyzing and planning on the fly, so this range of certainty helps us tend toward action.

When you try to achieve more than 70% information (or confidence, experience, etc.), your lack of speed can result in many negative consequences. It can also destroy your momentum or stem your interest, effectively meaning nothing's going to happen. There is a high likelihood of gaining nothing further from surpassing this threshold. Of course, most of us skew toward trying to attain 100% perfect information when we are dealing with fear and avoidance.

Let's say you're opening up a cocktail bar, which involves buying a lot of different types of liquor. You can't expect to have absolutely all the liquor you will ever need ready when the doors are ready to open. But on the other hand, it doesn't make sense to commence operations without enough for customers to choose from.

So you'd wait until you have at least 40% of available inventory. You've got momentum established. You figure if you could get more than half of what you need, you'll be in pretty good shape to open. You might not be able to make absolutely every drink in the bartender's guide, but you'll have enough on-hand to cover the staple drinks with a couple of variations. If you have around 50–60% inventory, you're probably ready. When the remaining inventory arrives, you'll already be in action and can just incorporate that new inventory into your offerings. If you waited until you had 70% or more inventory, you could find yourself stuck in neutral for longer than you wanted to be.

This way of thinking leads to more action than not. Waiting until you have 40% of what you need to make a move isn't a sedentary stay inside your comfort zone—you're actively planning what you need to do to get out, which is just fine (as long as it's not overplanning). Making the execution before you're 100%—or even halfway—ready to do so is the kind of gutsy move that lets you confront fear effectively.

Another way of looking at the math of fear is in the equation **fear = thinking + time.**

In this equation, fear cannot exist without thinking and time; take one of them away and there is no fear. For example, if you were offered a new position at work but would have to relocate to a new city, taking some time and giving it some thought should be expected. However, that time and thinking has to be limited in order to prevent you from thinking of new things to fear about making this decision.

If in researching the new city you were to discover a statistic showing there was a 2% increase in the murder rate from last year to this year, that might seem alarming. Then you would proceed to go down the rabbit hole and research how much of each type of crime there was in the past year, ultimately convincing yourself to stay put and not move. You had too much time, and fear was allowed to creep in via this equation. By giving yourself too much time and too much thinking, you have created more fear for yourself, and suddenly action may not be imminent.

Sometimes the parts of the equation are set by outside influences, like bosses needing to know decisions, but when you have the freedom, you now know how to reduce your fear. Just like a child standing at the candy counter trying to decide what to pick, by prolonging your decision, you prolong your wait to getting what you want.

The 40–70 rule does not take away thinking or time but limits them both. Nor does it take away the need for research or thoughtful consideration. Chances are, you are not going to work out the math when making decisions. However, what you *will* reach is the perception that you aren't gaining anything new from further procrastination. And that is when action is key.

A common obstacle faced when the 40–70 rule is met and it is time to take action is the thought "I still feel afraid." This is normal and expected and isn't a sign of not being ready. Separate fear and readiness. It is possible to feel terrified, have shaky hands or shallow breaths, and still take action. It does not matter one bit how you feel doing it; what matters is that you take the action.

Make Action Your Default

While limiting your thinking time can get the wheels turning, it's also important to think about how you typically respond when new situations arise. Your default is your go-to; it is what you do automatically. For people who struggle with allowing fear to keep them stuck, sometimes a change in their default is necessary.

For many, the original default is to do nothing or freeze or retreat. Sometimes, in an effort to fake action and feel somewhat productive, people will research and educate themselves right into inertia.

Research is important, but too many people get too caught up with the idea that their plan has to be perfect before it can go anywhere. Research does not have to be perfect; it does not even have to be that good. If a person is willing to take an action step and then respond to the feedback as she moves forward, that is far more valuable than more research.

Action is followed by two things: motivation and confidence. Once they take an action, people are motivated to see it through—it's out there, people know about it, and no one wants to look like a quitter. As success comes, people become more confident in themselves and in their decision to move forward. It becomes a glorious cycle of taking action, feeling motivated, gaining confidence, and repeating.

Making action the rule of thumb is one way to get out of the rut of overanalyzing and over-researching before making a decision. Unless there is a potential to cause real and permanent damage or pain, taking action and considering the consequences later is one way to live fearlessly. This is where you leap before you look.

After all, most of the time action will not result in any real damage. It may result in the need for a small apology; it may result in the need for a reversal; it may result in something that does not even matter in the long run. The fact is, sometimes, when taking action is the rule, you will succeed, and sometimes you will fail; when inaction is the rule, you always remain stuck.

One way to let action rule is to "lead with yes." Every time someone asks you to do something, as long as it is not dangerous or illegal, say yes.

Rock climbing? Yes. Salsa dancing? Yes. Sushi? Yes. Hiking the Grand Canyon? Yes. Kissing someone on top of the Empire State Building? Yes, if you can choose the someone.

Leading with yes is certainly one way to practice overcoming fears. Will you be embarrassed sometimes? Probably. Will you try some things you do not like? Chances are, yes. However, the more comfortable you get trying new things, the more motivated you become to try something else, the more confidence you gain, and we know how that cycle works to our advantage.

Excuses, Excuses

People use excuses to postpone taking action against fear. Most excuses, however, are poppycock—invalid, rubbish, and rationalized. Excuses are our subconscious protecting us from our fears. It is your automatic pilot saying, "Danger! This is going to be scary! Let me save you!" Let's look at some common excuses people use to postpone decision-making and facing fears.

Now is not the right time. True. There is never a perfect time for anything. There are mediocre times and terrible times, but rarely are there perfect times.

Timing is everything, except for telling a good joke—that's actually not true. Timing just *is*. There is no good time for a crisis, but they happen anyway. When attacking fears, rarely is there an obvious time that is better than another. It's just a lie we tell ourselves. There are always going to obstacles to overcome and hassles to manage. In fact, 99% of the time you want to do something, the timing will be mediocre, 1% the timing will be truly terrible, and that's it. There should never be any expectations of having perfect timing.

When is the right time to travel? When is the right time to get married? When is the right time to have a child? When is the right time to quit? You know the answer to these questions.

Selling a house is an excellent example. There is never a perfect time to sell a house. The housing market is never predictable, and various rates are subject to change overnight. You also don't know what bids you will receive and if anyone will even view your home. On the other hand, there are some objectively horrible times to sell a house, like when a main employer in town lays off 50% of its workforce and interest rates take a 10% rise.

Many of us wish timing was something we had more control over, but the fact remains, we rarely get to choose when something happens to us. We do, however, get to choose when we take action. Once you know what you need to know, the time to act has arrived.

I don't know where to start. You do; the problem is, you think you need an entire plan before starting. People need to stop expecting to see a clear path through to the end before they even begin.

Here is the secret: you don't need to know where you will finish to know where to start. The number one college major for students entering university in the U.S. is *undecided*. Most 18-year-olds are not able to articulate what they want to study that will lead to a life-long career. However, we encourage young people to get to college soon after high school. "Don't wait too long. Don't get too many responsibilities." During the four (or five) years they are on campus, most students declare a major and start working toward a degree that will eventually lead to employment.

We think nothing of this process; however, so many times in adulthood people become paralyzed because they don't see a clear finish line. Doing something today with what you have today is the key. Stop researching, stop agonizing, stop wasting time, and start doing. Do what you can do right now at this very moment, and you can figure out the next steps after. You probably know your next steps, however small they may be.

The blank page or the blank screen is the writer's nightmare. It does not matter if the writer is a middle schooler with a book report due or Stephen King. The blank page is terrifying. And yet, all who eventually produced something to fill that paper or screen had to stop reading the book, stop researching the topic, stop planning out the flow, and just start writing. The first words written may not be any good. They may be terrible and need to be changed. But the writer cannot get there if no words ever get down. The way to start writing is simple: start writing. Focusing on the end product, a hardback with a glossy cover, isn't the goal at the beginning. A beginning is the goal.

No matter what seems to be paralyzing you, use what you have in order to take action now. If you start working, you will soon see where you need to focus your attention and efforts. After you start, the rest will take care of itself because you will know what needs to be done to get you to the next step and then the one after that.

I'm not good enough. Shockingly, that just might be true. A person may really want to do something, but they might not be good enough. What is the answer to that dilemma? You can *become* good enough.

Sometimes the only way to get what you want is to shift into a growth mindset and start working. Make sure that, this time next year, you know more than you know now and that your skills are better than they are now. If you are willing to take the first steps, what you need will follow.

When you feel like you are not good enough, you might need to reframe it just a bit to "I'm not good enough at this moment." After all, why would anyone have the expectation that she would be good enough at something without practice, work, and a significant amount of time. You simply cannot have the expectation of instant or even preemptive excellence. If you never start, you will never be good enough, and you will have prophesized your own future.

Learning a musical instrument is an illustrative example. When people say they aren't musical before picking up an instrument, it makes little sense, does it? If learning to play the piano is your goal, then you can certainly make it happen. You would have to start back at that beginning Middle C, but with lessons, practice, patience, and perseverance. Anyone, including you, can learn to play the piano. Who knows? Perhaps you could eventually become a keyboard player for a Queen cover band. Just because you are not good enough now does not mean you cannot become good enough eventually.

Combating excuses is difficult because of our overwhelming need for self-protection. We may not even realize when we are using defense mechanisms to allow our fears to remain unimpeded.

But overcoming our fears requires action. We cannot think them away or research them away. Sometimes that means quitting a dead-end job or leaving a loveless relationship, while other times it means learning a new skill or honing an old one. Those things do not happen on their own. Someone has to act.

In Chapter 7, we will look at real, concrete action steps that allow people to overcome fear. Once you know what to do, then you have to take the first steps to move forward.

Takeaways:

- At some point, you can't simply talk your fears into disappearing. You can't reason with them, so in most instances, a little bit of action is required. This is best summed up by trying to embody fearlessness, which is ignoring the long process for confidence and just jumping into the deep end of the pool. Full confidence is difficult to attain, and you can accomplish more by acting fearlessly.
- The 40–70 rule is important for encouraging action because it accurately

portrays how much information you need. You need more than 40% of what you perceive you'd need, but no more than 70%. The problem is, most of us want 99% of information and certainty before we attempt something, and that just creates inertia.

- Fear = time + thinking. Remove one of those elements and you will feel less fear with every decision you come across. Again, thinking is good, and so is time, but only in moderation in regards to squashing fear. Make action your default mode of thought, and you'll get much further than you would otherwise.

- Most of your excuses against action are, in a word, fake. These include "now is not the right time" (there's never a perfect time), "I don't know where to start" (start with what you can do right now, not with an entire scheme created), and "I'm not good enough" (you might not be good enough at the moment, but you can get good enough).

Chapter 7. Anti-Fear Tactics

There has been a lot of talk about identifying fear, adjusting mindsets, and changing self-talk, but in order to overcome fears, people need actionable, real-life techniques to help them deal with and confront specific fears better.

This is a chapter of action, and as we saw in the previous chapter, action is what really matters most. As we come face to face with the real steps that can really help us overcome our fears, we must not allow ourselves to be trapped by overthinking, over-researching, or making excuses. Action must become our practice.

Embrace Your Feelings

In order to understand taking control of our fears, let's consider a research study conducted at the University of California, Los Angeles, on a group of people with a serious fear of spiders that they were hoping to overcome. To start the study, participants were divided into two groups and then put in the same room with a large, living tarantula.

They were asked to move as close as they could to the spider. The first group was told to verbalize their feelings and fears. As they moved closer and closer, they said things like "I'm scared. This thing is huge. It's so disgusting. I hate this." The second group, however, was told to keep quiet but to try to distract themselves while moving closer to the spider. Perhaps they tried to think about something else or concentrate on a spot on the floor. During the exercise, researchers measured things like pulse, breathing rates, and perspiration—all the physiological signs of fear. Later, each group was sent in to see the tarantula a second time.

Again, the same physiological changes were measured. This time, however, the first group, the ones who had verbalized their fears, was able to get much closer to the tarantula than the group that had simply tried to distract itself.

This tells us some important things about our fears and what helps us overcome them. First, it tells us that verbalizing our feelings about something we fear is important. Naming the problem, giving it an identity, and being honest about how that problem is essential in bringing that problem into perspective. Tarantulas are scary, but the reality is, they are spiders and at least 100 times smaller than a human being. They are destroyable with a single shoe.

As someone who is terrified of spiders comes closer to saying "It's just a spider" and having that mean "I can beat this" is a huge step. Why does this work? Because when you know what you're dealing with, you know how to cope with it better instead of feeling a general haze of *dread*. When you describe and label something, you are forced to do it in real, literal terms, and this tends to take some of the nightmarish mystique out of it. It makes it *real*—which is good, because otherwise it would be an unpleasant fantasy. You give yourself something tangible and concrete to deal with, which is easier to handle.

This study also tells us is that imagining something else, thinking about something else, or putting our head in the sand won't really help the situation at all. That second group was told to distract itself. We all have plenty of experience with that. We can distract ourselves with thinking and research and excuses and unlimited time and what-ifs until we have completely talked ourselves out of any action.

Distractions from our fear are also distractions from reaching our goals. Sitting on Facebook instead of going out with friends is not going to make you feel less lonely. It might distract you for a while, but in the end, you will still be sitting there with your phone, and maybe a dead battery, but nothing more to show for your time.

Our lesson from this study is to verbalize our fears and confront them head on if we want to overcome them. Ignoring them while secretly wishing they will go away on their own is not helpful. No matter the fears or phobias, this is the first step we can take toward eliminating them. It is unfortunate, but there's no secret path otherwise.

The next step to eliminating fear is learning that you can handle the discomfort it brings.

In order to illustrate this, let's conduct a quick experiment. Start by remembering a time when your anxiety level was extremely high. Try to recreate the physical reaction you experienced. Perhaps your heart was racing; perhaps your breathing was shallow; perhaps your stomach was in knots. Continue to think about that experience and try to recreate those same physical reactions. As you experience those uncomfortable feelings, try to increase the level of intensity as much as you can. As difficult as it may be, try to maintain the level of discomfort for about 10 minutes. Once the time has passed, you can bring yourself back to normal by controlling your breathing, walking around, or getting some water.

The point of this exercise is for you to realize that even when undergoing the full physical reaction to fear, you can manage it. Even if you were able to conjure up a full-blown panic attack, you survived it. You did not pass out or wet your pants or vomit. And even if you did do one of those things, that's all that happened. You still survived and life goes on. We are programmed to get through stressful situations. Learning to manage the uncomfortable physical and psychological responses when we are taking an action or when we are leading with yes is an exceptionally effective weapon in our fight against our fears.

The technique of imagining ourselves going through a painful or uncomfortable situation is not new. Samurai warriors trained themselves not to fear death in battle by using this same sort of visualization—in fact, they spent quite a bit of time ruminating on death because it gave them peace about constantly heading into battle.

As we imagine ourselves going through something that really scares us, experiencing the horrible feelings and surviving those feelings is empowering. It is almost like creating a vision board on Pinterest, only the vision isn't of the perfect wedding or an amazing kitchen—it is of yourself managing the things that terrify you.

Here is an example of how to start embracing your fears with the purpose of overcoming them. If you are someone who fears confrontation, start by naming it. "I am afraid of having a confrontation with a coworker. I am afraid it will get ugly and personal and our relationship will be destroyed." Naming the fear takes away its power and gives you a roadmap to beat it.

When we name it, it becomes "just" whatever—just a spider, just a discussion. It is really not the confrontation that is frightening, but rather the potential results of the confrontation that are frightening. Instead of focusing on the frightening confrontation, imagine your feelings if words get heated. It probably won't feel good, but you can discover that the feelings are manageable.

By imagining anxiety and controlling your physical and emotional reactions to that anxiety, you become more comfortable as the time for confrontation arises. It is just like with spiders. The participants in the research study did not stop having a reaction to the tarantula; they simply learned they could survive being a little uncomfortable in its presence. Learning that you can overcome a fear is truly powerful.

Face That Fear

After naming and embracing the presence of fear, it is time to face it with the intention of eliminating it.

If you recognize that you are afraid of embarrassing yourself in front of your friends, that's progress, but now you have to take the steps to get rid of that fear. If you admit you are afraid of dating because you are afraid you will get hurt again, you've named it, but if you want to be in a relationship with someone, you have to learn how to move past that fear of dating.

One reason we fear has to do with *fear-conditioned memories*. A person who had a near-drowning experience might start to feel anxiety any time she smells chlorinated water. She associates the smell of a swimming pool with the experience of choking, swallowing too much water, being unable to breath, panic. All of those feelings could return when she catches a whiff of that smell. Even though she is not drowning, the sensations associated with it are there.

In order to extinguish a fear-conditioned memory like that, you must face the fear-stimulus, but in a safe environment. So a patient might be placed in a completely safe, dry room but able to smell chlorinated water while having a pleasant experience like watching a home movie of a happy family event.

This new exposure needs to last long enough for the brain to form a new memory that conveys that the fear-conditioned stimulus is no longer dangerous in the present environment. This therapeutic approach is called *extinction*, and its results can be quite remarkable. You rewire your neural circuits to recognize that the stimulus is safe and no negative consequences will follow it.

Why does extinction work? Studies of brain images suggest that extinction may involve a strengthening of the capacity of the pre-frontal cortex (PFC) to inhibit amygdala-based fear responses (Phelps et al., 2004). Remember, it is in the amygdala that our brain experiences the most primary responses to fear. By retraining the brain to have a different and new automatic response to a certain fear stimulus, the fear can be eliminated.

Return to the example above about fearing confrontation with a coworker. After naming the fear, the next step is being exposed to the fear. This might be a good point to practice confrontation in a safe environment. You could ask someone to role-play and practice with you, or you could look for times when you could initiate a confrontation that is not really that big of a confrontation.

For example, if you order a meal at a restaurant and they bring you the wrong thing, it is not nitpicky to ask them to correct it. It is also good practice at standing up for yourself and confronting someone's mistake. And while no one likes a complainer, practicing in situations like this will let you learn that confrontation does not have to be rude or ugly. It will also help you learn that when you do have confrontations, there is almost always a way to work it out. This can ease anxiety when the confrontation is more serious or about something more important than mashed potatoes or cottage fries.

Exposure Therapy and Pushing the Comfort Zone

Exposure therapy is a form of cognitive behavioral therapy that involves subjecting patients to increasing amounts of the thing they fear or hope to avoid. This is the process of extinction taken to the extreme. Recall the examples above about the tarantula and the chlorinated water. By learning to become comfortable with the things most feared, most of the fear gets taken away.

Exposure therapy has been one of the great success stories of mental health techniques. It has done wonders for people with phobias, but it has also been a valuable treatment for other disorders as well. Research on cases of intense fear and traumatic brain injury has shown that, for a number of problems, the only way out is through.

In recent years, more attention has been brought to the issue of concussions, both in professional athletics and in child sports. And while concussions are quite common, we are just now learning how damaging they can be. For example, after a concussion, many people find themselves unable to work. Reading for any length of time kicks off bouts of dizziness. Bright light, including that from a screen, brings on crashing headaches. Even thinking can be completely exhausting. Many people just want to sit in a quiet dark place and enjoy zero mental stimulation.

Though the vast majority of concussion sufferers are fully recovered within three months, a "miserable minority," about 5%, have persistent and debilitating symptoms. This is when exposure therapy can really benefit a patient. By slowly reintroducing the patient to productivity, improvement can occur. For example, the patient may return to work by gradually increasing his time in the office or on the computer.

Starting with three to four hours and working up to an eight- or nine-hour workday helps the brain adjust. Similarly, physical movement can be added in increments. There is no need to run a marathon on your first day back at it. Taking time and slowly adding in more activities for a longer period of time allows the brain to tolerate more intense activities. Only by pushing through the misery, it seems, can the brain return to its normal activities.

Just as people can recover from concussions by gradually increasing their exposure to activities that require more and more brain power, others can reduce their adverse reactions to fear by gradually increasing exposure to the things they fear. It is based on the idea of classical conditioning (recall Pavlov and his salivating dogs). The therapy is conducted slowly by gradually increasing exposure to the things that are frightening. As the patient becomes more comfortable and relaxed with a frightening object, another more frightening object is presented. This goes on until fear is overcome.

Many people have an extreme fear of snakes. Treatment using exposure therapy might start with pictures a cartoonish-looking stuffed snake. After looking at the pictures he might be introduced to a real stuffed toy snake and eventually hold it. Over time, exposure would become more realistic. Going through the process of handling realistic-looking toy snakes to watching videos of real snakes to eventually being in the same room with a snake, the patient would slowly become able to control the emotional and physiological reactions he has toward snakes.

The science behind the success of exposure therapy is convincing. In order to understand how it works, let's consider a study out of Tufts University that was recently published in the journal *Neuron*. The report showed that exposure therapy remodels an inhibitory junction in amygdala, the fear processing center of the brain.

They knew that when mice were put in a fear-inducing situation, a small group of neurons in the amygdala was activated. What they discovered, though, was that when the mice had been exposed to fear-inducing situations gradually, like in exposure therapy, the neurons became less active. The reduced activity of the neurons decreases the chemical and biological response; therefore, the end result is a reduction of fear.

Burn Your Bridges

A common piece of advice we have all been given is not to burn any bridges. Generally speaking, that's sound advice. No one wants to go back to a former boss and have to take back some slanderous statement made in the exit interview or storm out of meeting only to remember the only way home is with the coworkers in your carpool.

Brett Kelly, however, suggests that sometimes we need to burn a few bridges to defeat fear. By finding a point that is difficult, or even impossible, to turn back from, you, in effect, have only one direction to move: forward. As a tool for overcoming fears, this one sounds a little frightening. The whole premise is to set yourself up to either prove you can do something or be stuck in a serious jam.

One of Kelly's examples is to buy a nonrefundable airline ticket to a place you've always wanted to go but have no idea how you will survive when you get there. Sound impossible? Consider Steve, a teacher at an international school, who always travels the exact same way. He books a ticket to one city and plans for three days' lodging and activities. He books his return flight from a different city, perhaps in the same country or perhaps in a bordering country, at least a week into the future. Then he spends three days in the first city and at least a week making his way to the second city.

Could you do it? Of course you could! Armed with a smart phone with a few travel apps like Trip Advisor and Google Maps, you would be totally fine. Admittedly, it would have been more difficult 20 years ago, but today it would be no different than going to a city an hour away from home.

What about a lesson from the conquests of Hernán Cortés, who was best known for conquering the mighty Aztec Empire in 1519. Well, he quite literally gave his men no choice by wrecking his ships onshore, thus ensuring that they would have to carry on, fight, and face a veritable army of angry natives.

Kelly is actually on to something that can be quite effective when it comes to taking action outside of your comfort zone. Fear keeps us stuck in the same old stagnant place. Putting yourself out there in new situations will force you to face a fear without turning back.

Just Breathe

Whether you're landing in a new city or walking into a bank to request a small business loan, breathing is always a good call during a stressful situation. There are many ways that practiced breathing can be really helpful. Margarita Tartakovsky, Psych Central editor, explains it this way: "Deep diaphragmatic breathing is a powerful anxiety-reducing technique because it activates the body's relaxation response." As psychologist Marla W. Deibler told Psych Central, "It helps the body go from the fight-or-flight response of the sympathetic nervous system to the relaxed response of the parasympathetic nervous system."

As a result of hundreds of thousands of years of evolution, we have developed knee-jerk reactions and neurochemical responses to stimulation that are often highly undesirable when it comes to performing optimally. As mentioned in previous chapters, the fight-or-flight response is one of these, which puts you into a state of massive physiological arousal and makes your mind go blank and all plans to fly out the door. These responses indeed contributed to increased chances of survival, but unfortunately, they don't have much of a place in modern society.

Being able to relax and focus in order to avoid distractions from natural stress responses is essential for sticking with your plan. Ordinary people simply can't control knee-jerk reactions such as shaking hands and sweaty palms because those reactions are caused by powerful hormones, including cortisol and adrenaline. We secrete hormones in large doses when we are under high stress or experiencing a good deal of fear, and controlling those secretions in the moment is next to impossible for us.

For Navy SEALs, however, succumbing to undesirable responses will mean the difference between life and death. As you might expect, they have some techniques that help them maintain clear mental states even in the most dangerous and stressful environments. One of those techniques that anybody can easily use is what's known as box breathing (Mark Divine). This means that when SEALs recognize that they are feeling overwhelmed, they regain control by focusing on their breath—breathing in for four seconds, holding for four seconds, exhaling for four seconds, and then repeating until you can feel your heart rate slow down and normalize. It is designed to calm the body down, because the mind tends to follow the body in times of potential crisis.

A stressed-out mind is an inefficient and uncreative mind, and so it is crucial for you to be able to remain calm if you want to perform to your full potential. Box breathing is simple to implement, and if it works for Navy SEALs, it can certainly work for us. The technique itself is easy, but the real key is to be able to recognize when your arousal might spiral out of control and sabotage your self-discipline.

Whenever you feel your heart beginning to race or your palms beginning to sweat, try focusing on your breath to reign in your undesirable reactions. If you can use box breathing at the first hint of physical arousal or stress, you will fare well because you will be able to control it. It's easier to stop it rather than manage it.

Meditation practices also often involve focusing on the breath and have a similar effect of reducing fight-or-flight instincts. However you go about it, controlling arousal can make a world of difference. Maybe it's the next time you're anxiously anticipating speaking in front of an audience or perhaps taking an intense and important exam. Whatever it is that causes you stress, you'll be more adept to handle it with a clear mental state.

Overall, just gain some perspective about fear. Consider the fable of the six blind men and the elephant.

Each is touching a different part of the elephant. One says he is touching a snake, one says he is touching a wall, one says he is touching a tree, one says he is touching rope, one says he is touching a fan, and one says he is touching a spear. None of them are right because none of them gets the big picture. Sometimes when we shift our focus, bring it out bit, or tighten it up a bit, we can see what we are dealing with. When you know exactly what you've got to work with, it makes tackling it a little less intimidating.

As a reader of this book, you need to decide which of these tools will work for you and how you can use them to overcome the fears that hinder you on a day-to-day basis. Most tools are easy to use on your own and can be modified to fit your specific needs. For example, you probably cannot effectively treat yourself with exposure therapy if you are dealing with the aftermath of a concussion or a debilitating fear of snakes.

You could, however, use some of its strategies to become more comfortable going out alone or having difficult conversations. By doing your own sort of "exposure therapy," you can take small steps to make you more comfortable doing something you fear. By practicing a series of deep-breathing exercises, you can learn to control your physiological responses to fear.

In the final chapter, you will go through a 21-day process to help you overcome the fears that hold you back. If you decide to stop reading now without completing the exercises, you will have new knowledge, but you will not have a new plan.

If you really want to have that formidoectomy, to cut the fears that hold you back out of your life once and for all, then you need to turn the page and take the steps. It will require some thought, some planning, and some action. There was never a promise of a magic wand or button. Please join in and change the way you face your fears.

Takeaways:

- This chapter is about some concrete, tangible methods you can use on your fears today. The first method is about embracing and labeling your fears. Presumably, when you can give a name to your fear and not run from it, you are forced to snap out of your nightmare and describe it in literal, unassuming terms. This takes your fears out of the ether and into a form that you can deal with on a logical level.

- A more action-oriented method is essentially facing your fears, but in a safe manner. This is to encourage extinction, which is when the negative feelings you have toward something extinguish. The more involved version of this is exposure therapy, where someone is gradually exposed to greater increments of what they fear. This works on the premise that, little by little, people acclimate to their fear and simply grow accustomed to fear because they have seen for themselves that no terrible consequences are associated with it.
- A more caustic method of dealing with fears is to burn your bridges behind you and force you to move forward and commit to action.
- A more introspective method of dealing with fears is to learn deep breathing techniques that Navy SEALs use to control their physical arousal and thus their reaction to fear.

Chapter 8. 21-Day Fear Action Plan

This chapter is designed for you to take everything from *Beat Fear* and formulate it into a concrete plan that will change your perception toward fear in general.

This plan is meant to take 21 days, though you may speed through some days and be stuck on others all the same. What's important is going through the sequence, no matter how long it takes.

The plan is conveniently split into three phases by week. The first week focuses on the mental aspects of fear, and that's where you take the time to think about what you fear and why. Thankfully, there is little to no action required here, just mental evaluation. The second week is a combination of further evaluation and baby steps of action. The third week puts all your introspection to work and actively seeks to tackle fear and wrestle it to the ground.

Week 1

This is your week to be thoughtful. Think about the things you fear, and be specific about them. Look back at Chapter 3 and consider the things that really frighten you or the things you avoid to the point they hold you back. Look at the examples and see how they compare to your experience.

Day 1: Fear of failure. Think of a time you wanted to do something but didn't because you were so were afraid of failing. An example might be something like learning to water-ski. Maybe your family spends two weeks at the lake every summer, and water-skiing is one of the highlights. Everyone seems to have so much fun, but you never learned how to do it. This year, you really want to join in, but you're afraid to try. What are the real fears in this scenario?

Are you truly afraid of physically hurting yourself? Or are there other barriers to taking action, such as a fear of judgment and looking foolish in front of family members and strangers?

Think about something you'd like to try but are afraid you might fail at. Take time to really consider all the ways you could fail. Then imagine what it would be like to succeed. Does it seem worth taking the chance?

Day 2: Fear of rejection. The fear of rejection is a legitimate fear. It's hardwired into our brains. No one wants to put themselves out there only to learn they aren't good enough. Everyone's experienced rejection in some way or another. Some of us feel we've never lived up to our parents' expectations, while others still feel traumatized by a middle school bully. Let's consider an example of someone who struggles with the fear of rejection as it relates to her work, which is creative in nature.

Jenny studied photography during her first two years of university, but she didn't finish her degree because of her financial situation. Five years later, she works for a company that produces school yearbooks, so she goes into schools in a four-state region to take photographs. When her cousin married last year and couldn't afford a professional photographer, Jenny stepped in, and the photos turned out great. She's interested in starting her own side business, but she's afraid that she just got lucky with her cousin and that her work wouldn't be in demand. She's also afraid that "real" photographers would laugh her out of the business.

Jenny fears rejection by potential clients and by other photographers. When you think about your own dreams and goals, who are you afraid would reject you? Think about how it would feel if instead of rejecting your ideas, people were excited about them. For that matter, how likely is rejection in reality versus the odds your imagination has created?

Day 3: Fear of judgment. The fear of judgment goes hand in hand with fear of failure and rejection. After all, in order to fail or be rejected, there has to be some sort of negative judgment on you. One common aspect of a fear of judgment is a fear of feeling embarrassed. The physical reaction of embarrassment—feeling hot, red cheeks, a racing pulse—is bad enough. Knowing that anyone who witnessed your snafu might be judging you amps up the level of discomfort.

Remember when Susan Boyle first stepped on the stage of *Britain's Got Talent?* If you don't, stop reading right now and pull the clip up on YouTube. Today's lesson can wait.

The judges on that show were judging her before she sang the first note of her song. Because of her looks, her dress, and her demeanor, they passed judgment instantly. Susan Boyle had to know that was coming. It's a talent show; there's an expectation that everyone is going to be judged. Yet she refused to let a fear of judgment stop her from trying. She went on to win the season and earned a recording contract.

Think about one of your dreams or goals that requires you to be like Susan Boyle, and step out and do something totally unexpected without fear of judgment. What would you have to do to take that step?

Day 4: Fear of change. So many life events are accompanied by change. Even when someone experiences a horrible situation, sometimes it feels safer to remain in the situation instead of risking a change. This is often the case with victims of domestic abuse. "If he's hurting you, why don't you just leave?"

It's a simple question with no easy answer. In part, leaving is so scary because it would bring massive change—in finances, housing, friends, status, etc. If children are in the picture, there could be school changes or daycare changes. Also, family and friends would change their attitudes about you and your spouse. All those changes are terrifying, and maybe you think that this is as good as it gets. Keeping things status quo, even if that includes walking on pins and needles most of the time, often feels easier and safer than making changes.

Consider something you'd like to do but would require major changes in your life. Think about the obstacles you'd need to remove—or at least set aside—for you to make that happen.

Day 5: Fear of the unknown. A big reason why change is so scary is because we never know what will happen next. Sometimes the devil we know is better than the devil we don't know. People often find themselves stuck, especially in their work. They really want out and to find a new job, but because they don't have a crystal ball that shows the future, they never venture out.

Recently, Zoe left her job of 14 years and took a similar job in a different city. Even though the nature of the work was similar, there were still many unknowns occupying her thoughts late at night. Being afraid of the unknown causes people to fear the big stuff and ask questions like, "Will I earn enough money? Am I qualified to do the work? Will I need a lot of training?" They also ask questions that almost seem trivial, like, "Who will I eat lunch with? Where will I park my car?"

Think about a time in your life when you had no idea what would happen next. Consider what *did* happen and how you managed the situation. Were you afraid of something, or were you just uncomfortable with the uncertainty?

Day 6: Fear of success. Recall the section about the fear of success, which told the story of Frank Abagnale. If you've never heard of him, stop reading and immediately research his story. His life story was made into a movie, and no matter how unrealistic it seemed, it was fairly accurate. For several years, he conned his way out of his shenanigans. When we feel like we're in over our heads, however, most of us don't have Frank's poise and confidence to get out the way he did.

We've all had moments when we felt like a fraud—not the perfect mom, not the perfect wife, not the perfect employee, not the perfect boss, not the perfect daughter, not the perfect friend, and so on. Guess what? No one expects you to be the perfect—except for maybe you.

Is there an area of your life where you feel like you're a fraud? Think about the ways you regularly demonstrate you can manage the demands of that role. Look at the hard evidence that defies your instinct to be fearful.

Day 7: Other fears. Go back and reread Chapter 4 about adjusting your mindset. Some of the ideas mentioned in that chapter might be new to you. Take some time today and do some research on the Stoics, Buddhism, and *amor fati*. Think about implementing some of those practices into your daily life. Take note on how they deal with fear and hardship with an attitude of "and then what?"

Summary. This week's activities have focused on the mental aspect of fear. Thinking about and naming some of your fears is the first step in learning how to deal with them. Keep these ideas in mind as you consider the fears you have focused on this week:

1. Fear is not bad. It has a real and valuable purpose.
2. Everyone, even those who seem most confident, struggle with fear from time to time.
3. When fear keeps you from being the person you want to be, find a way to overcome that fear.
4. Overcoming fear might not be easy, but it'll help you reach your potential.

Next week is a transition week. We'll remain focused on the thoughtful side of overcoming fear, but you'll start making plans for action. Having a good plan is one of the best ways to beat something you fear. By this time next week, you'll have plans in place to take real steps toward overcoming the fears that hold you back.

Week 2

This week is a combination week. You'll spend a lot of mental energy thinking about your fears, but you'll also apply this to real-life situations. This week, we're going to focus on Chapter 5 and apply what happened to you during the previous week. You're going to be writing some things down, so you'll need a journal of some sort to complete this week.

Day 8. Think about the previous week and list all the occasions when you experienced a fearful reaction. Your list should include both small, everyday things, like speaking up in a meeting at work, and big-picture things, like considering a new job. Don't judge yourself; simply make a list. It doesn't matter if fear kept you from stepping out and doing what you wanted or if you tried to overcome it but failed. If you really struggle with fear holding you back, your list could get quite lengthy, but that's not a problem. Remember, experiencing fear is normal. Be as detailed as possible.

Day 9. Chapter 5 focused on your inner monologue—those things you tell yourself. Go back to your list from yesterday and choose at least five fearful situations from last week. Try to recall what your inner voice was telling you when you experienced the fear. Write down some of the words you heard, either positive or negative, when you were going through those situations.

Day 10. Again, go back to that list from Day 8. This time, find examples on your list that could've been either fearful *or* exciting. Choose at least one event from your list that had the potential to be exciting but became a source of fear instead; in other words, choose a situation in which your inner monologue convinced you that caution (fear) was more important than experiencing excitement.

Write out what you inner monologue was saying when you were contemplating fear versus excitement. Now turn the situation upside-down and write out what your inner monologue *could* have said to convince you to choose excitement instead of fear. You can also try to change your inner monologue to something positive or reappraised. Talk to yourself differently and understand how to eliminate fear from the equation.

Day 11. Remember, fear has a purpose in our lives. It's our warning to be cautious. Too much of the time, though, we beat ourselves up for experiencing fear. Do you give yourself permission to experience fear, or do you use fear as another whip to beat yourself with? Fear is natural, and it doesn't become a problem until it prevents us from experiencing the life we want. Look back at your list and mark the fears that frustrated you the most.

Were you mad at yourself for not cold-calling a potential client? Do you wish you would've gone for coffee with your new neighbor across the hall? Identify those experiences where you let fear win instead of stepping out of your comfort zone for a new experience. You may have been turned off by fear but forgot that fear is neither negative nor evil.

Day 12. Reappraisal allows you to look at a situation in a new and fresh way. It gives you the opportunity to see something from a different perspective. Again, return to that list from Day 8. When did you experience a fear that was ripe for reappraisal? Perhaps it was when you let your mother's phone call go to voicemail because you were expecting her to nag at you about something. Perhaps it was when you avoided eye contact as your boss was looking for volunteers to head up a new project. In your journal, write about how you could have changed your inner monologue so that you could reappraise the situation. Be specific.

Could you have told yourself something that would've given you the courage to answer your mother's call or volunteer to take on something new? How can you eliminate fear from the equation?

Day 13. We're going to break down prudent versus fearful over the next two days. Today, consider a situation from your Day 8 list when you genuinely acted in a prudent manner. Choose an instance when it really was in your best interest to be prudent. Maybe it was in a meeting, when you were tempted to bring up someone else's mistake but kept it to yourself instead. Afterward, when you learned some additional facts about the incident, you realized that your coworker really had saved your department from a potentially costly error. Write down the inner monologue that convinced you to be prudent.

Day 14. Recall that even though it's easy to be prudent, often you're simply acting out of fear. Look back over your list and find an instance when you convinced yourself you were being prudent but were really using prudence as excuse to avoid moving forward on something. Maybe, for example, your sister called and invited you on a girls-only weekend trip. Even though it sounded fun and wasn't going to be expensive, you said no because you convinced yourself that the prudent thing to do would be staying home and catching up on some household chores. Write down what your inner monologue could have said to make you say yes instead of using prudence as your excuse to miss out on something.

Summary. Before we move on to Week 3, look back over the journaling you did this week. Do you see any patterns? What can you do to change your inner monologue so that you can examine the situations in your life in an objective manner? How can you start living a life motivated by curiosity rather than fear?

Week 3

This is the week you've been either waiting for or dreading. It's time to take some real action steps to help yourself learn to live fearlessly. This is not about eliminating all fear, but about learning to control your fears. You're going to practice the techniques mentioned in Chapters 6 and 7 and start using them in real situations that would normally cause you to respond in a fearful manner.

Day 15. Today, you'll start practicing the box breathing technique mentioned in Chapter 6. It's a four-count exercise that will allow you to control some of the physiological reactions to fear. Remember, on each step you'll count slowly to four in your head. Let's go over each of the steps.

Start in an upright, comfortable position and slowly exhale. Inhale slowly through your nose while counting to four. Hold your breath while counting to four. Exhale through your mouth while counting to four. Hold your breath while counting to four.

Repeat this process until you start to feel calm. If you like symmetry, try doing a series of four sets. Each day, repeat the series several times to help manage your feelings of fear or anxiety.

Day 16. Continue to practice your breathing technique, but today, you're going to take an action when you're only 70% certain of success. No more overthinking or overplanning. If you're reasonably certain you can achieve your desired outcome, then step over that threshold. This could be a real challenge for you. Your goal is to reach a point where your default setting is to act. For now, though, make sure you do it at least once today. If you get the opportunity to act more than once, go for it.

Day 17. Today's goal is to reduce the number of times you say no. You're going to attempt to lead with yes when an opportunity arises. The only time you can say no is if the opportunity is too expensive or if it's life-threatening. Eating lunch with coworkers instead of at your desk is not life-threatening; setting up an account on an online dating site is not outrageously expensive. Say yes, especially to things that are a bit out of your comfort zone and to things you've always secretly hoped to do. Additionally, shorten the time it takes to respond with yes. Don't waste time weighing the pros and cons or agonizing over the decision. Consider it, and then accept.

Day 18. Today, you're going to attempt to do your own version of exposure therapy. Don't worry, you don't have to lie down in a pit of snakes, but you do need to start spending time exposing yourself to something that makes you a bit uncomfortable. For example, many people are uncomfortable around animals. If your only experience with a dog included lots of jumping, drool, and perhaps even a nip, that's totally understandable. However, if you feel like your reaction to meeting a dog causes too much panic and anxiety and is negatively affecting your life, then you need to work on it. Going to a park where people walk their dogs would be a good way to start your own version of exposure therapy.

Consider the fears that send you into near-panic mode, and look for a way to have a very mild exposure today. Perhaps that's watching as cars safely drive over a bridge or finding a video about spiders.

Day 19. Play a little game with yourself when you face a fear today. If you're nervous about a presentation, add a little self-deprecating humor. If you're worried about a conversation with a friend, trust that, at any time, you can call time-out and start over. When something goes completely wrong, laugh about it and start fresh.

Day 20. Today, you're going to find a way to burn a bridge. Set yourself up to do something outside your comfort zone. Then manipulate the situation so that you can't get out of it. Uncomfortable taking public transportation? Have your spouse drop you off at work with no other way home. Nervous to meet your significant other's parents? Call them up and invite them to dinner (you don't have to cook). It doesn't matter what it is; just make sure you don't have a way out.

Day 21. Look back at the various techniques you've tried this week. Some may have been beneficial, like developing a practice of deep breathing, while others may have seemed extremely difficult, like burning some of those bridges. Think about which techniques were most effective. Don't think about the ones that were most comfortable; think about the ones that had the most positive results. Come up with likely life scenarios where you could use those techniques on a regular basis to help you gain control of your fears.

Summary. Now what? If you really believe that your fears have been holding you back and you honestly want to change that, you can't set this book back on the shelf or throw it in the donation bin. You need to take the advice offered here and work to make it an everyday, natural part of your life. Some of the tools and techniques are tried and true, and they could potentially help you make your desired changes. The only way that happens, though, is if you put them into practice.

You've read, you've analyzed, you've planned, and you've reviewed. Now take it to the next level, and take your life to the next level by working to make these techniques eliminate fear.

Summary Guide

Chapter 1. "Formidoectomy"

- Fear is not something we can control, even though it is one of the most basic human feelings. Fear may have had purposes in the past, but it seems like it only serves to keep us from what we desire these days.
- We fear *fear* more than anything else, and sometimes this is because we feel a lack of control. We may not always fear the actual consequences, but the uncertainty can be paralyzing. Therefore, it is best to stop fixating and creating an imagined nightmare in your head and focus on what is possible to control.
- Though we are all familiar with traumatic experiences and the toll they can have, sometimes we ignore how stress and anxiety can build up from daily reactions

199

to fear. They are just as important to deal with and shouldn't be overlooked.

- Dr. Karl Albrecht developed what he called a feararchy, which documented the five most prevalent and universal fears. They include extinction, mutilation, loss of autonomy, separation and rejection, and humiliation.

Chapter 2. The Origins of Fear

- Even though it seems that fear's only purpose is to keep us from what we want in life, fear has been one of the most powerful safeguards to life. This is because of how we respond to a fear stimulus: *freeze, fight, flight, or fright.* Biologically speaking, that is how your brain will process fear and cause you to act. Thus, much of what we want to accomplish in this book is to go against your ingrained instincts.
- There are two main pathways for fear: a primary and secondary pathway. The primary pathway is instantaneous and subconscious, and it is what triggers the three-step fear response. The secondary

pathway is slower and conscious, and it causes us to ask, "What is the problem here and how do I deal with it?"

- Fears are mostly instinctual, but they can also be learned and taught. These are no easier to shed.

- Despite the negatives of fear, it still has three important roles in our lives. If you care to listen and not react by fighting or fleeing, fear can act as your protector, motivator, and analyst.

Chapter 3. What Really Matters

- Even though we have gone through numerous models of fears, including Albrecht's feararchy, these are not necessarily what plague us in everyday life. The more realistic and tangible fears we are facing typically have to do with social constructs.

- Perhaps the most powerful fear we hold and live by is the fear of failure and rejection. This is powerful because it can create an effect where we wish to avoid failure and rejection; thus, we do nothing, because that gives us a 100% chance of avoiding that negative feeling. This is known as learned helplessness. The only solution here is to reframe how you view failure and rejection—it doesn't cause the end of the world, and it can be your best teacher.

- The second truly commonplace fear is the fear of judgment. This is another social fear. We care far too much what people think about us and let it dictate our decisions. We are skewed to believe that we are perpetually in the spotlight, which is patently untrue. We let this all affect our self-worth, which means we define ourselves by the perception of others, not ourselves. Often, a cost-benefit analysis will reveal that the fear of judgment is negligible, while the life you are missing out on is unfortunately massive.

- The third fear we face is the fear of change and the unknown. Like fear itself, change is neutral, but we always think about the worst-case scenario and fear that we are making a grave mistake. Attempt to switch your focus from all the possible obstacles to everything that is currently going right. If all else fails, find support and comfort in the factors of your life that won't ever change.

- The final fear we face is the fear of success, which sounds paradoxical. The truth is, many of us don't like the ancillary effects that success brings, such as increased attention and expectations. People don't want to be put under scrutiny and thus are prone to self-sabotage.

Chapter 4. Shift Your Mindset

- The mindset we have regarding fear can color our entire world. The perception of mindset as an important element of success was first proposed by Carol Dweck, who found differences between growth and fixed mindsets.
- As far as how it relates to fear, a mindset to avoid is the victim mentality. This is where you feel that you have no control about what's happening to you, and you necessarily view everything as a plot designed to bring you down. Obviously, this makes fear even worse because it feels inevitable and unstoppable.

- Another mindset to adjust is the inferiority complex, which is when you simply feel that you are not good enough or worthy of good things happening. This contributes to fear because it creates fear out of thin air, even when you should feel confident.

- A mindset to start embodying is *amor fati*, which translates to love of fate. When you can abide by this, you can embrace and love when something fearful or negative happens to you, recognizing that it is neutral and you can turn it into something positive—at the least, something neutral. You are not giving up or accepting mediocrity; you are simply moving past the present and thinking about how to proceed after the fact.

- A final mindset to learn is that of taking calculated risks. This is difficult in the face of fear because we can't help but think emotionally and irrationally. Thus, we ignore statistics and probabilities and make poor decisions. Attempt to remain even-keeled and objectively evaluate risk so the presence of fear isn't making you reactionary.

Chapter 5. Choose Your Inner Monologue

- Your inner monologue is the little voice inside your head that tells you to beware, be careful, and overall fear what comes your way. But, it can be changed. Your inner monologue doesn't have to take that angle—we should strive to improve it so it can empower us, not disempower us.

- The first way to change our inner monologues is to choose for the voice to dwell on excitement versus fear. Excitement and fear are often two sides of the same coin, but one of them promotes a positive attitude, while the other makes you cower and want to retreat.

- The second way to change our inner monologues is to give yourself permission to feel fear. The presence of fear is not a failure, nor it is uncommon. It is a natural part of any process. Therefore, if fear is present, take it as a sign that you are on the right path instead of the feeling that something is deeply wrong with you.

- The third way to change our inner monologues is to practice reappraisal, which is the act of framing a fearful act in a silver lining type of way. Studies have shown that simply relabeling something drastically changes how we feel about it, and we can do the same thing for fear.

- The fourth way to change our inner monologues is to choose prudence over fear. Instead of being fearful, you are being smart, cautious, and prudent. Again, when you harp on emotions other than fear, fear tends to fade. Just make sure this doesn't become a convenient excuse for yourself.

Chapter 6. The Case for Action

- At some point, you can't simply talk your fears into disappearing. You can't reason with them, so in most instances, a little bit of action is required. This is best summed up by trying to embody fearlessness, which is ignoring the long process for confidence and just jumping into the deep end of the pool. Full confidence is difficult to attain, and you can accomplish more by acting fearlessly.
- The 40–70 rule is important for encouraging action because it accurately

portrays how much information you need. You need more than 40% of what you perceive you'd need, but no more than 70%. The problem is, most of us want 99% of information and certainty before we attempt something, and that just creates inertia.

- Fear = time + thinking. Remove one of those elements and you will feel less fear with every decision you come across. Again, thinking is good, and so is time, but only in moderation in regards to squashing fear. Make action your default mode of thought, and you'll get much further than you would otherwise.

- Most of your excuses against action are, in a word, fake. These include "now is not the right time" (there's never a perfect time), "I don't know where to start" (start with what you can do right now, not with an entire scheme created), and "I'm not good enough" (you might not be good enough at the moment, but you can get good enough).

Chapter 7. Anti-Fear Tactics

- This chapter is about some concrete, tangible methods you can use on your fears today. The first method is about embracing and labeling your fears. Presumably, when you can give a name to your fear and not run from it, you are forced to snap out of your nightmare and describe it in literal, unassuming terms. This takes your fears out of the ether and into a form that you can deal with on a logical level.

- A more action-oriented method is essentially facing your fears, but in a safe manner. This is to encourage extinction, which is when the negative feelings you have toward something extinguish. The more involved version of this is exposure therapy, where someone is gradually exposed to greater increments of what they fear. This works on the premise that, little by little, people acclimate to their fear and simply grow accustomed to fear because they have seen for themselves that no terrible consequences are associated with it.

- A more caustic method of dealing with fears is to burn your bridges behind you

208

and force you to move forward and commit to action.

- A more introspective method of dealing with fears is to learn deep breathing techniques that Navy SEALs use to control their physical arousal and thus their reaction to fear.

Made in United States
North Haven, CT
03 September 2022

23633150R00117